TO BUY *or* NOT TO BUY ORGANIC

• ABOUT THE AUTHOR •

CINDY BURKE is the coauthor of *The Trans Fat Solution*, with *New York Times* food reporter Kim Severson. Burke writes about food, organic farming, and nutrition for numerous publications. Before working as a chef and food consultant, she studied at the school for American Chefs in Northern California's Napa Valley. She lives with her family in Seattle, Washington.

TO BUY *or* NOT TO BUY ORGANIC

• **ALSO BY CINDY BURKE** •
(with Kim Severson)

The Trans Fat Solution:
Cooking and Shopping to Eliminate the
Deadliest Fat from Your Diet

• CINDY BURKE •

TO BUY *or* NOT TO BUY ORGANIC

what you need to know
to choose the healthiest,
safest, most earth-friendly food

Marlowe & Company
New York

To Buy or Not to Buy Organic:
What You Need to Know to Choose the Healthiest,
Safest, Most Earth-Friendly Food

Published by
Marlowe & Company
An Imprint of Avalon Publishing Group, Incorporated
245 West 17th Street · 11th Floor
New York, NY 10011–5300

AVALON
publishing group incorporated

Library of Congress Cataloging-in-Publication Data

Burke, Cindy.
To buy or not to buy organic : what you need to know to choose the
healthiest, safest, most earth-friendly food / Cindy Burke.
p. cm.
Includes bibliographical references and index.
ISBN-13: 978-1-56924-268-1 (trade pbk.)
ISBN-10: 1-56924-268-2 (trade pbk.)
1. Natural foods—Health aspects—United States.
2. Natural foods—Economic aspects—United States.
3. Grocery shopping—United States.
4. Consumer behavior—United States. I. Title.
TX369.B87 2007
641.5'63--dc22
2006101822

9   8   7   6   5   4   3

Designed by Pauline Neuwirth, Neuwirth & Associates, Inc.
Printed in the United States of America

To my mom,
who loved her grandmother's farm.

We haven't got the power to destroy the planet—or to save it.
But we might have the power to save ourselves.

—Ian Malcolm,
character from Michael Crichton's Jurassic Park

• contents •

. . . .

• introduction •

Before I started writing this book, I thought I already knew the answer to the question *To Buy or Not to Buy Organic?* I've been a food writer since the 1980s, and have also worked as a cook, a chef, and at an organic food home-delivery service. I've been buying organic food for many years, and my young daughter rarely eats any food that isn't organic. So I thought the obvious answer to that question was . . . buy organic!

I was surprised to find out that the answer isn't so simple anymore. When I talked with growers at my neighborhood farmers market, several of them told me that their farms were no longer certified organic. I was shocked. What had made these growers decide to use pesticides after years of being "certified organic?" Oh no, they told me. They would never use pesticides on their farm, or give hormones and antibiotics to their animals. These farmers were still growing food the way they always had, but they had decided that the cost and bureaucracy of being a certified organic grower was no longer worth it. When I talked with farmers in Ohio, Oregon, Washington, New York, Louisiana, and other areas, I heard similar stories.

Many of the farmers I spoke with have been farming organically for ten, twenty, or even thirty or more years, and they are worried about where the organic marketplace is going. Many of the same evils to which organics were supposed to provide an alternative—monoculture, low wages, dependence on fossil fuel, industrial farming structures—have been reincarnated as the big-business version of "certified organic."

Some were disgusted with the attempts by agribusiness lobbyists to persuade the government to weaken organic standards, so they had decertified their farm in protest. Others saw that large growing operations were taking over the organics marketplace and eroding their profitability, so they couldn't afford the certification process.

Still others were immigrants from Mexico, Laos, or Vietnam, and did not have sufficient language skills to fill out the required paperwork. And some, well, some were just plain ticked off that in order to be certified organic, they had to provide government inspectors with full access to their farms, their accounting records, and their strategy plans, when they believed the farms that needed monitoring were the conventional farms.

Yet there are still plenty of dedicated farmers who take pride in growing certified organic food and livestock. These farmers say that the "certified organic" label is the only way for consumers to be certain that synthetic pesticides are never used on their food.

As I talked with other people about how they made decisions on what food to buy, a few things became clear. We all want to make food choices that improve our quality of life. But it was equally clear that sorting through the issues involved as to where we shop and what we eat was confusing to almost everyone, including me. Concern about the effects from pesticides had led me to select organics almost exclusively. Because I was seeking healthier, safer food choices, I felt that organics were the only way to know for certain that my food was chemical-free.

But organic food can be so expensive and difficult to find that I always wondered if I was spending my money and time wisely. Once I actually spent eleven dollars on an organic cauliflower—and then wondered the entire way home if that purchase was excessive and foolish. Swapping one kind of anxiety (over the risky effects of pesticides) for another (over wasting money at the grocery store) didn't feel like a good trade to me.

I decided to become informed, really informed, about the options—organic, conventional, local, sustainable—so that I could choose the healthiest, safest food available. Although I loved the idea of supporting local farmers, I often wondered which path was best—grocery stores, farmers' markets, driving to the farm, an organic home-delivery service, or even ordering through the Internet—so I looked into those alternatives as well.

I'm not a nutritionist. I'm not a scientist. I don't have any research organization, government bureaucracy, or corporation behind me putting words on these pages. I am a real consumer, much like you, who has a busy life and a family to cook for every day. I am aware that the food choices I make not only affect my health, my longevity, and my environment in profound and long-lasting ways, but they affect *your* health, *your* longevity, and *your* environment as well. We all live on the same planet, so it's worth taking the time to understand the options.

As I discovered, buying organic *is* a valuable measure you can take to eat healthier food, but it is not the only factor worth considering. Organics are actually starting to smell like yesterday's news, while local, sustainable food is becoming the fresh choice for **ethical eaters**. How do you sort it all out and still get dinner on the table? I've tried to examine and clarify the current issues about what kind of food to eat and where to buy that food. This book is primarily a guide to help you make healthy and cost-effective food choices.

No discussion of farming, especially organic farming, is complete without touching on the rampant use of pesticides and the alarming load of agricultural chemicals you and I carry in our bodies. Concerns about pesticides have brought many of us to organics in an effort to make healthier, safer food choices. Current scientific research is focusing on a new area of concern—pesticides and chemicals that are endocrine (hormone) disruptors. Chapter 2, " How Pesticide Exposure Impacts Your Health," reviews some of the current research about pesticides and the permanent health effects from even minuscule exposures.

The evolution of organics (some might say the rise and fall) is an intriguing story of an anti-industrial utopia created by farmers and hippies, embraced by consumers looking for safer food choices, and ultimately taken over by business and government. I could write another book exclusively on this subject (and several authors have), but this is not that book. Chapter 3, "Growing Organic Foods," will give you a basic understanding of the forces and events that created conventional farming and the backlash against it, which led to organic practices and standards.

I had the great pleasure of talking with people from all over America about organics and sustainable farming. Farmers, along with the people who order, sell, and deliver your food to you, and those who support those efforts, were important sources of information for me. They answered many questions and shared their expertise and experience. The profiles throughout the book are a closer look at some of the interesting conversations we had about organics, sustainable growing, life on a farm, the value of community, and many other topics. Throughout this book I emphasize the importance of getting to know the people who bring your food to you. I'm convinced—and I hope you will be, too—that there is no better way to be certain the food you are buying is clean and healthy. These profiles will help you to see how interesting it is to talk (or tromp around a cornfield or pasture) with the people who are responsible for producing your food. I hope you'll be inspired to strike up a conversation of your own with such people.

Chapters 5, 6, and 7, along with the summarized Shopping Guide (see page 157), provide detailed information about how specific foods are grown and *why* certain chemicals are used, or not used, on our food. Please note that when I offer you advice about whether or not buying organic is a wise choice, I am not just giving you my personal opinion. I spent a great deal of time researching farming practices, looking into pesticide data, reading agriculture reports from various universities, surfing the Internet, and conducting a number of in-depth conversations with farmers about how food is grown or raised.

Once you're ready to start shopping, you can find stores and other sources for healthy, safe, earth-friendly foods in chapter 8, "Where to Find Healthy Food."

If you see an unfamiliar word or phrase in bold type as you are reading, you'll find its definition in the glossary at the back of the book.

You'll also find resources at the end of the book that you can use to gather more information about organic, local, and sustainable food, as well as where to find it.

Make sure to bring along the Shopping Guide (see page 157) when you head out to the grocery store. This quick reference guide gives you advice on whether or not you should buy the organic version of more than one hundred common foods.

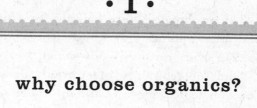

· 1 ·

why choose organics?

*I*N RECENT years, consumers in the United States and other countries have become more health conscious, more sophisticated, and more choosy when it comes to the food they eat. During 2005:

* Nearly two-thirds of American shoppers bought at least one organic food product.[1]
* Purchases of organic grocery items increased by nearly 15 percent as compared to 2004.[2]
* Organic food sales in the United States hit $13.8 billion in 2005, up from $11.9 billion in 2004 and a mere $3.6 billion in 1997.[3]
* Latinos and African Americans were the fastest-growing group of organic "core consumers."[4]
* In Canada, the number of certified organic processors more than doubled between 2003 and 2005, with the largest increases observed in

British Columbia and Quebec. Organically-
raised chickens flocks increased by a 56 percent,
and organically-raised beef herds increased by 30
percent.

Many of these shoppers were looking for a little extra
insurance. Just as antilock brakes and airbags on your car
make you feel safer, organic foods—which lack the scary
chemicals and biotechnology of conventionally farmed
food—allow you to feel more confident about your food
choices.

Americans have lived through many food safety scares.
Remember spinach tainted with E. coli? The presence of
rBST growth hormones in milk? Apples sprayed with the **carcinogenic** pesticide Alar? **Mad cow disease? DDT?**

Incidents such as these may pass fairly quickly through your
consumer consciousness and then fade away, but they have left
many of us looking for food that is safer and healthier. It's that
hunger for safer food, along with weariness from constantly
hearing about toxic substances in our food, that has caused
consumer demand for organic foods to explode over the past
eight years.

Common reasons that consumers give for choosing organic
food are:

* To avoid pesticides in their food and in their body
* To avoid the synthetic hormones found in milk,
  dairy, and meat (especially in the diet of their
  children)[5]
* To avoid the antibiotics commonly used in large
  feedlots and factory farms[6]
* To preserve the environment
* To support small farmers[7]

Selling the "Certified Organic" Sticker

Organic food offers you a greater peace of mind about your food. As the marketing strategists would say: you're not buying an organic peach; you're buying the opportunity to eat a peach without worrying.

That's a twisted way to look at it, but think about it. You know instinctively that it can't be good for your body to eat foods sprayed with insecticides and other toxic chemicals. You might also feel strongly that releasing these chemicals into the air, earth, and water is bad for wildlife, bad for the planet, and bad for future generations. So what do you do? You buy organic. But do you know for certain that organic foods are the better choice?

The **Environmental Protection Agency (EPA)** and **United States Department of Agriculture (USDA)** regularly tell American consumers that our conventionally grown food is the safest in the world. The EPA says that pesticide levels for conventional fruits and vegetables are allowed only in amounts that the agency has deemed "safe levels."

The growing market for organics seems to indicate that consumers just aren't buying that line of reasoning. After years of state-enforced standards (more about this in chapter 3) for organics, in 2002 the U.S. government decided it was time to take over. At that time, the USDA created minimum standards for foods labeled organic, and they began regulating the organic certification process and organic marketing. Now only produce that is from a "certified" organic farm or food processor can legally be sold as organic.

The official seal of USDA-certified organic foods is recognized by many shoppers. You've probably picked one of those annoying little stickers out of your stir-fry or off an apple skin. Although you may be a little fuzzy on exactly what that seal stands for, you probably assume that at a minimum it means the food was grown without synthetic pesticides or chemicals. So if a food doesn't have that sticker, I wondered, does it mean that it's always grown *with* chemicals and pesticides? Should I buy organic or nonorganic?

On every trip to the grocery store, that decision is revisited dozens of times. Organic or nonorganic? Select the cheaper apples or the organic apples? Buy the organic strawberries, or skip the strawberries entirely? Head to the farmers' market to buy local produce, or buy organic produce at the grocery store that has been imported from Mexico, Chile, and Australia?

WHICH GRAPES SHOULD YOU BUY?

There you stand in the produce aisle of your local grocery. In one hand you're holding a bag of conventionally farmed red grapes. In the other hand you have a bag of organically grown red grapes. Both look firm and juicy, and both provide vitamins and nutrition. The organic grapes cost more, possibly almost twice as much. And the organic grapes have a little sticker that says "Certified Organic" or "USDA Organic." Which grapes should you buy?

The choice you ultimately make may depend on the price difference. It might be determined by who's going to eat the grapes—you, your child, or your co-workers. You might pull off a grape from each bunch and see which one tastes better. Maybe that would be the easiest way to make your decision.

Now let's assume the organic grapes come from Argentina, and the nonorganic grapes are grown within one hundred miles of your home. Is it more important to support local growers and your local economy, and thus reduce the amount of fuel used to transport your groceries? Or is it more beneficial to buy organic no matter where that food was grown and how much fossil fuel was needed to get it into your grocery cart? Which grapes do you buy now?

That is the dilemma that is presently rocking the organics market. Organic doesn't mean local. Organic doesn't mean that any less fossil fuel is consumed to bring a product to market. Organic used to imply that your food was grown on a small family farm, but that is no longer true, either. And food can be both "local" and "organic" without being "**sustainable**." (See chapter 5 for more information about sustainable farming.) As Gene Kahn, who sold his organic company, Cascadian Farm, to Welch's (now a division of General Mills), put it, "We're part of the food industry now."[8] And while it has made some people very rich, the fact that organics are part of the food industry now has made other people very angry.

Lucy Goodman, a sustainable farmer in Eaton, Ohio (see the profile of Boulder Belt Eco-Farm, on page 6), says, "When the UDSA took over organic certification, it allowed the big players to market organics, and a lot of them have the same old attitudes. You know, they are making organic Twinkies essentially. They're doing whatever they have to do to slap the organic label on their products, because it's become a buzzword."

Boulder Belt Eco-Farm

LUCY GOODMAN *is a sustainable farmer with a lot to say. If you catch her on a rainy, cold winter night when there's not much to do on the farm, she will talk about almost everything—life on her farm, why some people don't cook, raising chickens, making ketchup from scratch, daytime television.*

Funny, inspiring, and insightful at the same time, Lucy is a passionate farmer who owns and farms Boulder Belt Eco-Farm near Eaton, Ohio, with her husband, Eugene. She sells her veggies, herbs, produce, chickens, and seedlings from her roadside farm store and at the Saturday farmers' market in the nearby college town of Oxford. She was a certified organic farmer for many years. Now she runs her farm as a sustainable "organic" farm without organic certification. That's because . . . well, let Lucy tell the story.

"For a long time, we were one of the few organic farms in this part of Ohio. I suspect the organic foods movement was seen as a backwater run by hippies and thus not taken seriously. Now that the hippies are raking in some cash, the multinationals think it is time to take over.

"In October of 2002, I voluntarily dropped my organic certification. That was after the USDA took over the process. I knew that no good would ever come of that! I've never regretted that move.

"When the USDA took over organic certification, it allowed the big players to market organics, and a lot of them have the same old attitudes. You know, they are making organic Twinkies essentially. If anyone thinks the USDA does a good job at oversight, take a look at the feedlot beef industry and all the problems there. Fast Food Nation is a great book on that subject."[9]

Although Lucy has not changed her philosophy about using agricultural chemicals (she's generally against it), soil balance (she thinks the USDA should stay out of her compost), or high-fructose corn syrup (she hates it), she has changed the way she markets her products. She's finished with jumping through hoops to gain organic certification.

"I have put in hundreds of hours trying to preserve the integrity of organics. I have written my reps in Congress. I have educated people about the importance of organic foods. I have complained to the USDA when they tried to weaken the standards. And yet the corporatization of organics continues," she says with a sigh.

"I am busy. I have a lot of crops to plant and harvest, and markets to go to, and, you know, I just don't have the time or energy for this fight any longer. Instead, I put my efforts into promoting local agriculture and educating people on the importance of supporting local farms over organic corporations."

So Lucy and Eugene continue to farm without chemicals and without the distribution options that can come from being a certified organic grower. Instead of relying on what she sees as a dubious government stamp of approval, she relies on regular contact with her customer network. During the growing season she sends weekly e-mail updates to her customers to let them know what's available that week. Her e-mails are a lot like a conversation with her—filled with stories of life on the farm, her philosophy of life, and details about the food they grow on the farm.

Here's an excerpt:

> **Watermelons**—We still have a few Yellow Doll melons, not much else, but hey, it was a wonderful melon season and all good things must come to an end!
>
> **Tomatoes**—We still have some really nice 'maters—from the big red hybrids to our homebred striped tomato (yes, we are amateur tomato breeders, and our new cultivar is very, very tasty).
>
> **Strawberries**—from our ever-bearing plants. Excellent sweet flavor, no pesticides, and out of season. Who else has fresh homegrown berries, I ask you?

Lucy and Eugene encourage their customers to come out to the farm, take a look around, and see with their own eyes how they grow food at Boulder Belt Eco-Farm. She's happy—very happy—to talk with customers about their farming practices, why sustainable farming is better than organic farming, why pastured livestock is healthier, and why her 'maters and 'taters taste so good.

Lucy also writes a blog about Boulder Belt Eco-Farm, agricultural politics, farm life, and whatever else she has stuck in her craw that day. During those long, cold Ohio winters she often offers advice through several farm discussion boards to *novice and experienced farmers who want to try farming without pesticides or chemicals.*

She loves her farm, she loves talking to people who care about food and the environment, and in her own quirky way, she's changing the way people shop for food in her little corner of rural Ohio.

BOULDER BELT ECO-FARM
3257 U.S. ROUTE 127 NORTH
Eaton, OH 45320
http://www.boulderbeltfarm.com
http://boulerbelt.blogspot.com

THE MYTH OF THE SMALL FAMILY FARM

Shoppers often imagine that when they buy organic produce at the grocery store they are helping small family farms, but that is not necessarily true. When you peek behind the curtain (or read the label closely), you will see that it's often just business as usual for American food processors. Look at who really owns the companies in the organics industry, and you'll see a lot of familiar names:

Cascadian Farms, Muir Glen	General Mills
Morningstar Farms, Kashi	Kellogg
Back to Nature, Boca Burgers	Kraft
Odwalla	Coca-Cola
Seeds of Change	M&M/Mars
Silk, White Wave, Alta Dena, Horizon	Dean
Ben & Jerry's, Ragu Organic	Unilever
Knudsen Juices	Smucker's

Although there are a few large organic producers who vow to stay true to traditional organic ideology, such as the Organic Valley Family of Farms (see Resources), the organic grocery segment is now largely controlled by all of the same old players. Giving consumers the option to choose food grown without synthetic pesticides is a great concept, but these companies are not changing the way farms grow, produce, or sell food, because to do so would put them at a serious competitive disadvantage.

ORGANICS:
NOT WHAT THEY USED TO BE

Instead of organics changing the world for the better, it seems that, sadly, the world is changing organics. **Monoculture**, or growing a single crop (see page 36); heavy machinery; and trucking food thousands of miles to the grocery store have become the new norm for organic food production. *The New Yorker* quoted an unnamed consumer advocate as saying, "Organic is becoming what we hoped it would be an alternative to."[10]

To meet the growing demand for organic foods, the scale of organic farming has become massive. In 2006 the nation's largest retailer, Wal-Mart, announced that it would be doubling the number of organic foods items in four hundred of its stores. Many other grocery chains, such as Safeway, Kroger, SuperValu, Trader Joe's, and Whole Foods, are creating their own store-brand organic products. These changes in the organic marketplace will certainly increase competition and may drive prices downward (see page 51). And when prices go down, companies start looking for ways to increase production, outsource raw ingredients, and lower costs. So buyer beware.

One way that some organic food producers have tried to cut corners is to lower the minimum standards for organic products. The integrity of the "certified organic" label, regulated by the **National Organic Program (NOP)**, has been threatened several times by agricultural lobbyists. Consumers have been vigilant and beaten back efforts to weaken the standards, but the lobbyists keep trying to allow **GMO (genetically modified organism)** seeds, **sewer sludge,** and feedlot conditions to become legal organic standards.

THE "CERTIFIED ORGANIC" STICKER IS JUST A SUBSTITUTE FOR TRUST

The distance between people and farms has created a disconnect between the farmer and the consumer that didn't used to exist. The "certified organic" label is simply a substitute for knowing and trusting the farmer who grows your food. If you have a relationship with that farmer, if you see her every week at the farmers' market, you can just ask her if she uses pesticides on her raspberries or fertilizer on her lettuce. If you trust your farmer (or your store's produce buyer), you don't necessarily need to have a sticker on your food letting you know that a government inspector thinks it's free of pesticides.

Values are important, and farmers' markets are great. But on most days, convenience has the advantage over idealism. When you're on your way home from work, the farmers' market is not convenient, and you're simply looking for something to make for dinner, you may be likely to just stop in at the nearest chain grocery store. You may not even think your decisions matter very much, but they do.

In just over twenty years organics have evolved from "rabbit food" to a product category that a majority of Americans have in their home.[11] That change did not come about because big **agribusinesses** were concerned about pesticide poisoning, or because corporations suddenly started caring about the environment. No supermarket chain or megastore decided on its own that selling organics would be healthier for its customers.

That change in the marketplace came about because people—people just like you—changed their purchasing habits and started asking for healthier choices. After you read the next chapter, which covers new research on the effects of even tiny amounts of pesticides on humans, you'll understand why carefully considering your food choices is so important.

· 2 ·

how pesticide exposure impacts your health

IF YOU eat food in the United States, you eat pesticides. The **Food and Drug Administration (FDA)** estimates that twenty pounds of pesticides are used per person per year in the United States. At least *fifty* of these pesticides are classified as carcinogenic. In fact, there is a common term for using pesticides, herbicides, insecticides, fungicides, and other chemicals on food grown for human consumption—it's called conventional farming. Conventional, as in, that's the way we normally grow food in the United States.

I was surprised to learn that our government's intent is not to limit human exposure to toxic chemicals in our food—even for known or suspected human carcinogens like the **organophosphates** (pesticides, herbicides, fungicides) that are used on many conventionally grown foods. That would be bad for business.

Instead, the EPA conducts a cost-benefit assessment for pesticides. They register or license very toxic pesticides or livestock feed additives for use in the U.S., such as **methyl**

bromide and arsenic, when the chemical's potential economic benefit is deemed to outweigh the potential hazard to humans or the environment. Why does this not comfort me? Since the chemical and agribusiness companies have powerful, highly paid lobbyists (some of whom are former EPA employees) to pressure the EPA to keep chemicals on the market, many suspected human carcinogens or **endocrine disruptors** are *still* registered for use on food for humans and livestock. The EPA almost never bans a pesticide that is presently in use. Call me a cynic, but I also have just a tinge of suspicion that the U.S. government doesn't value my health nearly as much as I do. I also recall that our government told us that chemicals like DDT, thalidomide, and asbestos were safe . . . right up to the day the EPA banned them.

After looking into how things are done at the EPA, I feel even less confident in the agency's ability to protect the public from toxic chemicals in our food. For example, instead of completely banning a toxic pesticide, the EPA is more likely to merely restrict the application of a pesticide to specific times during a crop's growth cycle. That means it's up each farmer to monitor correct usage of the pesticide. If some farmer didn't get the memo, well, hey, what can you do?

In the rare instance where a ban seems inevitable, the manufacturer will often make an agreement with the EPA to take the chemical off of the market in the United States so that they can avoid bad publicity and preserve the option to market it overseas. There are virtually no deterrents to exporting pesticides banned or unregistered in the U.S. Pesticide manufacturers spend years of research and millions of dollars before seeking EPA approval and registration. If pesticides are not approved, manufacturers export them to Third World countries where restrictions on pesticide use are more lax. As you'll read in chapter 4, "Organic Economics," food in the United States comes from around the globe, so shipping carcinogenic pesticides overseas does not protect you from eating food sprayed with banned or unregistered pesticides.

New pesticides must now meet stricter health and safety standards because of the 1996 **Food Quality Protection Act (FQPA)**, but, again, it is rare for the EPA to completely ban a pesticide. Changes to EPA regulations are perpetually held up by complex scientific debates, which delay policy changes and keep pesticides and toxic chemicals on your food.

STRONGER BUGS AND WEAKER HUMANS

While researching this book, I spent several rather disheartening months reading studies about pesticides—arsenic levels in chicken, **persistent organic pollutants (POP)** in breast milk, pesticide-related hormone disruptions, mutations in aquatic creatures living downstream from cattle ranches, links between hormones in dairy cows and early sexual maturation in preteen girls.

I had to wonder: what are these toxic chemicals in our food doing to our bodies, and to our children's bodies? Parkinson's disease, heart disease, infertility, reproductive disorders, cancers, birth defects, learning disabilities—all of these have been linked with exposure to agricultural pesticides. By using so many pesticides and toxic chemicals on our food, we seem to be creating stronger bugs while creating weaker humans.

Like those cabbage farmers whose eyes were finally opened by the resilience of a moth (see page 4), many Americans are finally starting to catch on, too: *pesticides are not the solution.* Pesticides are a temporary fix to a systemic problem—that problem being that food cultivation has been transformed from an innovative, fruitful relationship between a farmer and a community into a factory-like system where only inputs and outputs are measured.

How Bad Can Pesticides Be?

Organophosphates may sound like a strange chemical compound, something only a laboratory would have access to, but you are probably carrying some of them around in your body right now. And here's the really scary part: they're one of the most toxic chemical compounds around, classified as a **neurotoxin,** carcinogen, and generally nasty poison.

If organophosphates are so bad, why do you have them in your body? They're commonly used in agricultural insecticides and as a result are found in trace amounts in many nonorganic fruits and vegetables. They're also found in animal feed, and thus in nonorganic animal products, particularly those with a high fat content, such as whole milk, butter, and cheese.

Because organophosphate residues are stored in fat tissue, they remain in your body for a long time. One of the most chilling pieces of information I read (in *Our Stolen Future,* by Theo Coborn, Dianne Dumanoski, and John Peterson Myers) while researching this book is that the most efficient method for ridding the body of organophosphates and other chemical residues is through breastfeeding. Nursing babies literally drain the toxins right out of their mother's body in breast milk.[1] Some scientists think this conveyance may be the reason why researchers have found that the more children a woman breastfed, the less likely she is to develop breast cancer.

In July 2006 BBC news reported comments from Professor Richard Sharpe, of the Medical Research Council's Human Reproductive Sciences Unit in Edinburgh, supporting that theory. Sharpe said:

> *The older the woman before her first breastfeeding episode and the longer and the higher her DDT exposure has been, the greater will be the amount of chemical delivered to the baby.*
>
> *So the first baby gets the worst of the chemicals stored in the mum's*

fat. There may also be a bonus to the mum in that she is ridding her-self and her fat tissue of the chemicals in question and because some of these chemicals are potentially implicated in the development of breast cancer—the breast is mainly fat.

This could be one of the ways in which early breastfeeding protects some mothers against breast cancer.[2]

ENDOCRINE DISRUPTORS MAY BE EVEN WORSE

As bad as organophosphates are, there is another class of chemical toxins sprayed on human food that are thought to be much worse. The endocrine (hormone) system is very sensitive to pesticide exposure, and over the past ten years scientists have done extensive research into studying how toxic chemicals disrupt endocrine signaling and function.

Pesticides are thought to interfere with normal endocrine signaling and function, and many pesticides are now considered "endocrine disruptors." That term is something of a catchphrase for chemicals that cause a variety of changes in normal hormone signaling.

Some better known examples of endocrine-disrupting pesticides found in foods are:

* DDT, an insecticide
* Vinclozolin, a commonly used fungicide
* Atrazine, an herbicide
* Endosulfan, a DDT relative with xenoestrogenic properties (those that imitate or increase the effects of estrogen)

One thing you should realize is that humans are never exposed to only one xenoestrogenic chemical. We are all exposed to multiple sources for xenoestrogens at the same time. Especially troubling is the fact that endocrine disruptors have been found to have an additive effect—that is, each new exposure magnifies the effect of every previous exposure. This additive effect is why extremely low potency and low concentrations of xenoestrogens can still cause significant hormonal disruption.

Although many scientists concur that pesticides can have life-changing effects on essential hormone signals in the human body, there is little agreement about how much endocrine disruption is too much, and how much, if any, is harmless.

DIFFICULTIES IN LINKING HUMAN HEALTH WOES TO PESTICIDES

The more scientists learn about the toxicity of pesticides, the more questions are raised about the potential effects on people. An often quoted statistic is that the EPA speculates that 60 percent of all herbicides, 90 percent of all fungicides, and 30 percent of all insecticides contain potential cancer-causing chemicals.[3] Yet the chemicals are still registered for use on food. Why? Pesticide manufacturers try to portray "no conclusive evidence of harm to humans" as an assurance of safety. The current regulatory system in the United States assumes that chemicals are not harmful until they are proven otherwise. To me, this naive presumption of safety allows your health and the health of your children to be put at risk.

There are three major reasons why it is nearly impossible for researchers to irrefutably link pesticides to human harm:

1. **Pesticides are too dangerous to be tested directly on humans.** Statements like, "We've found no conclusive evidence of harm to humans from exposure to pesticides" are created to mislead you into thinking that human exposure to pesticides, fungicides, and

other chemicals has been tested and found to be without risk. In fact, there is no testing of pesticides on humans (except accidentally, if it is found that registered EPA agricultural chemicals pose unacceptable health risks to humans). For example, even though studies on the effects of the pesticide endosulfan in animals suggest that long-term exposure can damage the kidneys, testes, liver, and may affect the immune system, it is still registered for agricultural use in the United States.

2. **Because people are contaminated with trace levels of hundreds, or even thousands, of chemicals, it is impossible to attribute a specific health effect to any one chemical.** There are a few exceptions, however— certain chemicals, like **PCBs**, and **heavy metals**, such as lead, are known to have permanent adverse effects on learning and behavior from low doses during vulnerable periods of growth.

3. **Most safety tests done for regulatory agencies like the FDA are not intended to determine if low-dose exposure to pesticides is safe.** Fredrick Vom Saal, professor of biological sciences at the University of Missouri, and a leading researcher in the field of developmental biology, explained in a 1998 interview with the PBS newsmagazine *Frontline* why he does not trust the current regulatory system: "The problem is that all chemical screening is controlled by industry hiring contract labs to screen those chemicals . . . [the data] goes directly to corporations through their legal departments. And then they decide whether to provide it to the government or not. They decide whether the outcomes are adverse. That could be very subjective, and they just say, 'Well, we didn't provide this information, because we didn't think it was a problem.'"[4]

HOW PESTICIDE EXPOSURE IMPACTS YOUR HEALTH

How Organophosphates
Do Their Deadly Deed

ᘒ

ORGANOPHOSPHATES ARE the lethal ingredient in many pesticides that are highly toxic to insects, birds, and mammals. Malathion, Dursban, and Diazinon are some common brand names of organophosphate pesticides. They have a chemical characteristic that leads them to dissipate very slowly once they are introduced to the body.

Why don't organophosphates seem to affect a farmworker spraying field crops? The Web site called "How Stuff Works" says the key is lethal dosage. A dose of organophosphate that would be fatal to an aphid is below the quantity that would have a noticeable effect on humans. Lethal dosages are based on weight, so when the dosage increases to a high enough level, an organophosphate-based pesticide that kills insects will harm humans as well. The Web site goes on to say that is why people are warned to keep pets and children off of the lawn right after treatment with a pesticide. Because children and pets have lower body weights than adults, and they inhale air much closer to the ground, they could receive a dose of insecticide sufficient to cause harmful effects. Organophosphate pesticides do their deadly work by attacking signals in the brain. Quickly absorbed through the skin, the chemical interrupts the electrochemical process that some **synapses** use to pass signals between nerve cells. The synapse provides the route for the central nervous system to connect to and control other bodily systems.

In a normally operating synapse, **acetylcholine** fires a signal between one neuron and another, or between a muscle receptor and a nerve. Then **cholinesterase** binds to the acetylcholine, which allows the nerve to have a rest between synapses. Exposure to an organophosphate prevents the cholinesterase from inactivating the acetylcholine. The effect is that messages sent by the brain cannot shoot across the synapses. The acetylcholine quickly builds up, and the muscles become overstimulated, leading to jerky movements, convulsions, paralysis, and even death. If you are a bug—or if you are human exposed to high enough levels of organophosphates—the onset of such symptoms may occur very rapidly.

Small doses of organophosphates can cause an inability to concentrate, or mild paralysis, or diseases of the heart and respiratory system. Evidence that even low levels of exposure to organophosphates are harmful to humans has been building for years.

* "How Does Dursban Work?" http://science.howstuffworks.com/question440.htm.

CHILDREN ARE AT A MUCH
HIGHER RISK FROM PESTICIDES

The government only mandates, and chemical manufacturers conduct, high-dose studies designed to find obvious toxic effects. Contract labs are hired to feed pesticides to rats until the rats die, and then they record that amount of pesticide exposure as being toxic. The model used to quantify these results is a 154-pound male adult. (For example, 760 mg of a chemical fed to a rat weighing 500 grams is considered equal to approximately 0.2 pound of the same chemical ingested by a 154-lb (70 kg) person. If rats begin to show toxic effects from 760 mg of that chemical, then the allowable level for humans would be set below 0.2 lb for that same chemical.)

Children, especially infants and toddlers, eat more food per pound of body weight than adults do. And as any parent can testify, they eat a much less varied diet than adults. This is why exposure to any pesticide from food is greater when quantified per pound of a child's body weight as compared with the effect upon an adult.

A "safe" level of pesticide residue for a 154-pound adult male is not likely to be safe for a small child. As an example, nonorganic strawberries typically contain multiple pesticide residues, including several suspected carcinogens. A typical serving for an adult would be one cup, or about one-half pint. Anyone with a child knows it is not unusual for a toddler, weighing in at about twenty pounds (including a wet diaper), to eat an entire pint of strawberries in one sitting. Not only do the kids ingest more pesticide per pound of their body weight, but also their physiology is much more vulnerable to damage from pesticide exposure.

The body of an infant or child is fundamentally different from that of an adult, and their organs continue to grow and mature from conception throughout childhood. In addition to the endocrine system, organ systems, such as the brain and nervous system, can be permanently, albeit subtly, damaged by exposure to toxic substances that at the same level would cause no detectable harm to adults.

Babies and Small Children May Be Exposed during Critical Developmental Periods

Beyond the narrow scope of government agencies, independently funded scientists have been researching the subtle ways that small doses of pesticides can have long-lasting adverse effects. Scientists have consistently found that the *timing* of the exposure is at least as important as the dose. During critical periods of fetal development and childhood growth, the fetus, infant, and small child are very vulnerable to the effects from even tiny amounts of pesticides and toxic chemicals.

Professor Vom Saal has researched the effects of low doses of natural and synthetic hormones on animals. His studies have shown that extremely low doses of hormones can permanently alter development of the reproductive system in mice (humans and mice share 99 percent of the same genes) and can cause irreversible changes that do not manifest until later in life. Vom Saal's research documents that ingesting low doses at a vulnerable moment of development can cause a more significant effect than high doses during adulthood.[5]

You read that correctly—a small dose at a critical moment in a child's development can have a more deleterious effect than a higher dose during adulthood. That is the reason why mothers-to-be are wise to try to eat pesticide-free foods during pregnancy and while nursing their baby. Scientist Vom Saal further explains why he thinks that traditional testing methods for suspected endocrine disruptors are obsolete. "[These methods] are based on the assumption that you can test massive amounts of these chemicals in animals and then predict the effects of the very low doses that we are exposed to. That is a false model. You cannot anticipate a low dose effect from a very high dose effect. Anybody who is trained in endocrinology or neurobiology knows that doesn't work for chemicals that communicate between cells like hormones or neurotransmitters, because high doses shut down the response system. Every doctor knows that and uses it clinically (for example, contraceptive pills which boost estrogen levels to stop ovulation). So you actually block responses at high doses while low doses stimulate response."

Pesticides in an expectant mother's bloodstream are definitely passed to her baby. In a 2005 study the umbilical cord blood of ten randomly selected newborns was collected by the Red Cross and tested extensively for contaminants. The Red Cross researchers found that 287 commercial chemicals, pesticides, and pollutants crossed the placental barrier. Among these substances were 21 different pesticides.[6]

Recent research has also produced strong evidence that exposing a fetus to low levels of organophosphate pesticides can result in babies with a smaller than normal head circumference, a known risk factor for reduced intelligence and behavior disturbances.[7]

It's Not Too Late to Make Changes

If your children are eating conventionally grown food, there's good news for you. Recent evidence shows that switching to organics can still be beneficial to children's health, even if they've already been exposed to pesticides. A study of this hypothesis was initiated by the EPA after a University of Washington researcher in a previous study (measuring dialkyl phosphate, or DAP, metabolites [the common breakdown products of organophosphorus pesticides] in children's urine) noticed that the pesticide level of one child out of the ninety-six children in the study was zero. According to the study, "[The] child's parents . . . reported buying exclusively organic produce and did not use any pesticides at home. This child was the only subject whose urine samples showed no measurable concentrations of any of the DAP metabolites."[8]

This discovery led to another study, this one published in 2005, which measured DAP in the urine of twenty-three children before and after switching to a diet of all organic foods. After five straight days on the exclusively organic diet, researchers found that pesticide levels in the children's urine had decreased to undetectable levels, and remained that way until the children returned to eating conventionally grown foods. The study's conclusion was obvious: "An organic diet provides a dramatic and immediate protective effect" against pesticide exposure in children.[9]

BLIND GENERALS LEAD THE WAR ON PESTICIDES

Scientists know that pesticides can change critical hormone signals in the human body in ways, such as infertility, that have life-altering effects. Yet in the absence of tests conducted at lower doses, pesticide manufacturers claim safety, because harm to humans has not been conclusively verified.

In *Our Stolen Future* authors Theo Coborn, Dianne Dumanoski, and John Peterson Myers note: "Like generals, pesticide regulators are always and perhaps inevitably fighting the last war. Again and again, they have vetted chemicals for the most recently recognized hazard only to be blindsided by dangers they never thought to anticipate. They judged DDT by the hazards of the previous generation of pesticides—the acutely toxic arsenic compounds that could bring sudden death . . .

Only after DDT had been spread as liberally as talcum powder across the face of the Earth did we realize that DDT brought death as well, but in a different way."[10]

Here is one very significant area where government regulation lags behind scientific research. Inert ingredients may make up more than 99 percent of the total pesticide formulation and may be significantly more toxic than the active ingredient. The **Federal Insecticide, Fungicide, and Rodenticide Act of 1972** only requires that manufacturers list the active ingredients on the label. The inert ingredients are considered a trade secret, and any possible dangers are not regulated. Many of the inert ingredients for pesticides are known to be "hazardous," "suspected carcinogens," and "extremely hazardous."[11]

Some of the active ingredients in common pesticides are chlorothalonil, a probable human carcinogen; piperonyl butoxide, which is toxic to the liver and a possible human carcinogen; dichlorvos, an organophosphate that can cause respiratory distress and paralysis; and chloropicrin, which has been linked to asthma and pulmonary edema. Inert ingredients in pesticides are not regulated or listed anywhere on the product label, nor, of course, on the food it is sprayed on.

INEFFECTIVE AND
WEAK GOVERNMENT

Oversight efforts of the U.S. government to monitor and prevent human exposure to chemical contaminants in the food supply are fundamentally weak for a number of reasons, but in part because accountability is fragmented between the EPA, the FDA, and the USDA.

Here's a summary of what each of these government agencies is responsible for when it comes to pesticides:

* The EPA determines whether a pesticide can be registered and approved for use and establishes the "tolerance level" for each chemical.
* The FDA enforces pesticide tolerances for all domestically produced food and imported foods (except for meat, poultry, and eggs, which are enforced by the USDA).
* The USDA is responsible for conducting random tests of fresh food for pesticide residues.

Instead of requiring that any chemical used on food pose *no* health hazard to humans, the agencies establish the "tolerance level" for food-use chemicals. A tolerance level is the maximum amount of a chemical legally permitted in food for human consumption. As long as a given chemical's residues fall below the tolerance level the EPA, FDA, or USDA have determined acceptable, conventional farmers can use those registered chemicals on food crops. To monitor compliance, the agencies annually test samples of produce, meat, dairy products, and eggs. The agencies have the power to pull food from the market if tolerance levels are exceeded, but that almost never happens.

The EPA especially is mired in constant political pressure and remains very closely aligned with chemical industry interests. Many former EPA officials go to work as lobbyists for the pesticide and agricultural companies after leaving the agency. Now former pesticide executives are even finding work within the offices of the EPA. A former pesticide-manufacturing executive for Dow Chemical and Arysta Life-Science was named to take over the Seattle office of the EPA in October 2006.[12] Appointing former pesticide-manufacturing executives to lead an organization called the Environmental *Protection* Agency may seem counterintuitive, but that's how our government chooses to "protect" our food supply and our environment.

Hepworth Farms

AMY HEPWORTH *knows her apples.* She and her family have farmed in New York's Hudson Valley since 1818, growing more than thirty varieties of apples. She and her family have been propagating, eating, and harvesting apples for her entire life.

She calls her apples "minimally treated," and she sells bushels of them. Amy is passionate about many aspects of agriculture, but apples and tree fruit are her main focus. She has a degree from Cornell University in pomology (fruit cultivation), and she understands the ecosystem of an apple orchard like few people do.

While attending Cornell in the late 1970s, Amy met others who were interested in creating alternatives to the chemically intensive farming methods that were common during that time. She recalls that the idea of growing organically was considered so bizarre that one professor refused to even grade her term paper about creating a functional five-acre organic farm. She had to take her paper to the school's dean to have it considered.

After her Cornell experience, she began experimenting at Hepworth Farms with the idea of growing apples organically. As she recalls, one day she decided that she had to "dechemicalize" her farm. "I just stopped spraying my trees altogether. I eliminated all herbicides from the farm, and I learned about how complementary plants and insects worked on a farm," she said.

How did that work out? "We lost crop after crop," Amy

recalls. "I would watch a Red Delicious orchard, and when the mites took over, the entire orchard turned brown and all of the fruit dropped on the ground.

"But what happened next was that the predators came in. It just took a little while for those bad boys to clean up the mites, but the mites had to get out of control first. You have to live with that cycle, and you have to tolerate some imperfection."

Hepworth Farms orchards now have a kind of wild peace—the insects, the weeds, and the birds all live in and around the apple trees, and Amy uses few, if any, chemicals. She believes the reason pesticide use became so rampant in the first place is that consumers are intolerant of even small blemishes or spots on fresh produce. "Farmers don't want to spray," she says. "It costs money, and it takes time. They would rather put up with a little black spot or a few aphids and spray less often, but consumers won't let them."

She now uses the least amount of pesticide possible, refusing to spray until she sees a large pest outbreak. Even then, she says, she will only spray an orchard twice at the very most. If two sprays are not sufficient, she simply lets the insects take the fruit and hopes the predatory insects and birds will clean up the pests next season.

Amy feels strongly that the apples from Hepworth Farms are the best they can be. She sees no reason to change her farming practices to make her apples certified organic. Even organic growers often spray their fruit to reduce pests and mites, according to Amy, using use nonsynthetic pesticides, such as sulphur, or using biological controls.

The farm does grow forty-five acres of certified organic vegetables that she wholesales to the Park Slope Food Co-op (see the profile on page 59) in Brooklyn, New York, and other stores, including Whole Foods. She became certified because the co-op insisted upon it, but says that growing organically "is not the most creative way to farm. It's not hard to do, but it's not creative.

"We live in a feel-good society; we're do-gooders—Americans especially. People want to do good, and they want to do something that is good for themselves," Amy says. "People have just caught on to the organics, as if that is the solution. If they were supporting the grassroots organic farmers, like back in the seventies, they would have gotten a superior product. Now when they buy organics, it's a gamble whether they are really getting something better.

"I think the movement of buying locally is the wave of the future. People who live in our town, or who come to our farm, are attached to our farm. They consider our farm to be their farm."

HEPWORTH FARMS
1635 RT 9W
Milton, NY 12547
(845) 795–2141

A Plague of Lobbyists

Here's even more evidence that pesticide manufacturer lobbyists affect government policies. In 2006 union representatives of the EPA's own scientists sent a letter to agency administrator Stephen Johnson complaining that they were being "besieged" by demands from agriculture and chemical company interests to extend the licenses of more than twenty pesticides thought to disrupt brain development in unborn babies and children. Primarily organophosphates and **carbamates**, the pesticides in question are linked with childhood leukemia and aplastic anemia, as well as non-Hodgkin's lymphoma, leukemia, and lung cancer in adults. They are also known to cause hormonal changes, DNA damage, birth defects, and abnormal sperm, ovaries, and eggs. These scientists warned Johnson that the EPA "may underestimate the risk to infants and children" of these toxic chemicals used in agricultural settings. The fact that the EPA is even considering extending the licenses for these chemicals to be applied to food is appalling.

The May 24 letter to Johnson, which was signed by nine presidents of EPA unions representing scientists and risk assessors, said, "We are concerned that the agency has lost sight of its regulatory responsibilities in trying to reach consensus with those that it regulates." You think? It seems to me that the EPA seems to be more focused on ensuring that distribution channels for chemicals remain open than they are on ensuring the safety of our food supply.

Changes to EPA regulations are slowed to the point of inertia by complex scientific debates and bureaucracy, and clearly the pesticide manufacturers like it that way. According to the 2006 letter referenced above, "Equally alarming is the belief among managers in the **Pesticide and Toxics Program** that regulatory decisions should only be made after reaching full consensus with the regulated pesticide and chemicals industry."[13]

Imagine sitting in a conference room, trying to reach an agreement with pesticide manufacturers to ban chemicals that make them millions of dollars in profit each year. It's never going to happen. Consensus building with pesticide interests only benefits them by delaying policy changes and keeping pesticides in your food.

WHO CAN YOU TRUST
WHEN IT COMES TO REGULATING PESTICIDES?

If you can't rely on the government to protect your interest, you have to be well informed and proactive. You know, I know—we all know—that pesticides, herbicides, and fungicides are highly poisonous. They are designed to kill—insects, weeds, fungus, rodents, and other "pests"—and that is the only reason the government regulates them at all. Our fragmented and weak regulatory system falls short of convincing me that the food grown by conventional farmers does not pose a danger to human health. I've talked with farmers who assure me that most farmers do not want to use pesticides if they don't have to, but I've also talked with several others who used to be conventional farmers and they say that several preventive sprays of pesticide and herbicide is still the standard.

I do know that known **mutagens** and carcinogens are still permitted in human food as long as chemical lobbyists convince the regulators that there is an economic benefit gained by applying these chemicals to food crops. I do not believe that the current regulatory system has been effective in protecting us from pesticides and other chemical residues in our food. The fact that methyl bromide (the EPA's own Web site calls it "highly toxic") is still allowed on strawberry crops demonstrates that we cannot entrust our food safety to these regulatory agencies.

WHAT CAN YOU DO TO PROTECT YOURSELF?

By now you should realize that you can't just blindly trust the EPA to look out for your best interests. Consumers are wise to try to find a direct route to organic and sustainable farmers.

Just as we make changes in politics with our votes, we make changes in products with our purchases. Building local food production routes, buying from farmers who grow food responsibly, and bypassing conventional food distribution are sure paths to healthier food. And as evidenced by the masses who are turning to organics, more and more of you are concerned enough about food safety to make changes in your shopping habits.

You have to protect yourself and your family. How can you do that?

1. You have the right to know what's in your food. Tell your grocer, farmer, or other supplier that you prefer to buy food grown without pesticides or other toxic chemicals. Ask them to post information on the pesticides and chemicals that are used on the food they sell. Ask them to post information about where the food they sell was grown and how far it traveled to get to you.

2. Realize that there are health risks from many pesticides used on food, especially for men and women who plan to have children, pregnant women, babies, and young children. Senior citizens and people who have a weakened immune system may also be at risk. If you or people in your family fall into these categories, be

very careful about choosing your food. Food grown without pesticides is the best choice to keep your body healthy and free of disease in the future.

3. For what it's worth, let the decision makers in our government know you do not want pesticides and other toxins on your food. Contact your congressional representatives and tell them to call for a ban on toxic pesticides in our food supply. Pester the heck out of them.

4. Write or e-mail the USDA and let them know that you strongly oppose any attempts to lower the existing organic standards. Stay informed about attempts to water down the National Organic Program (NOP) standards (see page 45).

5. Use the Internet to monitor and comment on FDA and EPA regulatory activities on toxic pesticides and other food additives through their Web sites. The FDA and the EPA take comments from the public before they make most decisions about changing regulations for food and animal food. Typically their offices are flooded with statements from chemical and livestock producers who want to keep using chemicals, antibiotics, and hormones in your food.

6. Meanwhile, choose food that is either organic, sustainably grown, or grown without pesticides, fungicides, synthetic fertilizers, or other toxins (see page 149 for more information about available options).

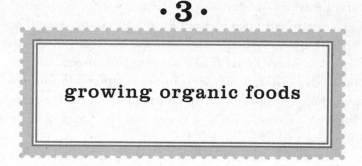

· 3 ·

growing organic foods

AFTER MONTHS of researching pesticides for this book and plowing through studies with titles like "Organophosphates and Head Circumference in Newborns"[1] and "Chlorpyrifos Factsheet: Human Exposure,"[2] I began to wonder what in the world made farmers think that spraying deadly bug killers on human food was a good idea. For most of human history there was no other way to farm *but* organically. Although organics are now being marketed as the progressive way to grow food, sustainable, chemical-free farming was actually the norm for thousands of years. The story of how farming changed from being a natural ecosystem—managed by a farmer and his family—to the modern factory farm system of inputs and outputs is worth knowing. Chemicals do increase the bushels per acre, making farms more profitable, but chemicals also create a load of other problems.

OLD-SCHOOL PEST CONTROL:
SAFER WAYS OF HANDLING THE PROBLEM

Back in the day, farmers controlled weeds and diseases by rotating crops and farming in harmony with the weather. They controlled mice and moles with predatory cats. They picked bugs off by hand and stomped on them or doused them with tobacco juice. The reality was that insects, rodents, and birds needed to eat, too—and there were a lot more of them than there were humans. Farmers simply had to accept that losing crops to pests, disease, and bad weather was an inevitable part of farming.

Prior to the 1930s most farmers grew just enough food to support their families and to occasionally sell or barter the excess to neighbors. Insecticides were largely unknown, because massive insect outbreaks were rare and isolated incidents. Some chemicals were around to control weeds, but they were not very effective and, in the midst of the Great Depression, few farmers could afford them.

It was only after the United States became involved in World War II that farmers made significant changes in the way they grew food. As farmers and their sons left to join the war effort, the era of horse- and mule-drawn plows came to an end. Tractors and heavy machinery performed tasks like plowing and weeding, which had occupied a farmer's entire family for many days.

A BUG'S-EYE VIEW OF MONOCULTURE

As more people moved to urban areas to work in wartime factories, farmers began to see an opportunity. Suddenly, growing large amounts of just one crop and transporting it by rail to the cities could be profitable. As rural farmers moved toward monoculture—that is, cultivating a single crop, such as wheat, corn, or soybeans—immense fields of identical crops soon spread out for miles and miles.

Farmers weren't the only creature to see an incredible opportunity in monoculture. Think about monoculture, for a moment, from the perspective of a bug. Miles and miles of identical fields providing a never-ending feast—it was hog heaven for hordes of hungry insects. With plenty of food clustered in one location, the insects had no reason to leave. Insects seized the opportunity of monoculture and quickly multiplied. By the early 1940s farmers needed a problem solver to eliminate insect infestations. At around the same time, U.S. chemical manufacturers needed a new marketplace for postwar chemicals.

EARLY PESTICIDE DEVELOPMENT:
FROM THE BATTLEFIELD TO THE BARNYARD

DDT seemed to be the perfect solution for both parties. Used during World War II to prevent common diseases carried by insects, such as typhus and malaria, DDT was issued to U.S. soldiers, who were instructed to sprinkle it in their clothing and sleeping bags. The success of DDT in controlling insect-borne diseases and saving the lives of thousands of soldiers led many to think of DDT as a miracle chemical. When the war ended, DDT and other pesticides were marketed to farmers. Most people assumed DDT posed no risk to human health, as the seemingly healthy returning war veterans appeared to demonstrate.

Farmers were eager to take advantage of this new miracle chemical to control insects in their fields, and widely embraced the new chemical pesticides and herbicides. Unfortunately, no one realized that the effects of DDT were much more insidious and far-reaching. Despite mounting evidence about the dangers of DDT and its propensity to accumulate in the food chain, the EPA allowed DDT to be a registered agricultural pesticide for over twenty years. After Rachel Carson published *Silent Spring*, documenting the link between DDT and cancer, the chemical was finally banned in 1972. (See "The American Public Contemplates *Silent Spring*" on page 41). DDT was only the beginning of the long-standing and current practice by the U.S. government of allowing chemical manufacturers to sell potentially toxic poisons to farmers with minimal testing on their impact to human health or the environment.

J. I. RODALE:
A PIONEER IN ORGANIC FARMING

Of course, there were always farmers who recognized the value of farming in harmony with nature, without pesticides. J. I. Rodale was a Pennsylvania farmer who was passionate about nurturing the health of the soil on farmlands. He was an early proponent of sustainable agriculture and organics, and started the Rodale Press, which published *Organic Farming and Gardening* magazine during the 1940s.

Rodale was one of the first Americans to publicly warn farmers against buying into the enthusiasm for synthesized chemical fertilizers and pesticides. "Organics is not a fad," he wrote in 1954. "It has been a long-established practice—much more firmly grounded than the current chemical flair. Present agricultural practices are leading us downhill."

Today the Rodale Institute, run by Rodale's grandson, still works to inform farmers and consumers about the benefits of organic and sustainable growth methods. Their goal is simple: "To put people in control of what they eat."[3] The institute's New Farm forums (see Resources) also offer advice and support for farmers who are transitioning to organics by connecting them to experienced organic and sustainable farmers.

The Cascade Harvest Coalition

THE CASCADE *Harvest Coalition works to build a sustainable regional food system in western Washington State. The coalition sponsors a number of events and programs to bring farmers and the surrounding community closer together. Mary Embleton has been the executive director of the coalition since 1999.*

She spent part of her life on her family's farm in Montana. "I think there are a lot of lessons that people can take away by connecting with a farm," she says. "When you become a member of a CSA [Community Supported Agriculture, see page 145], or you buy food at the farmers market, you're putting a face on the person that raises your food. It ties you to the community."

The Cascade Harvest Coalition now counts more than 150 farms, farmers' markets, schools, and other agriculture businesses as members. When the coalition first formed in the late 1990s, the founders brainstormed about what a perfect world would look like. When she pictures a perfect world, this is what Mary sees: "Lots more local production, with healthy, viable farms. People would be aware of the implications of their food choices, not only on their communities, but on the environment."

Mary works to help farmers stay afloat financially, and that often involves doing other things besides harvesting crops to increase visibility and make money. One of the newer trends for small farms is agritourism, which involves creating entertainment to bring people out to the farm. Agritourism activities include wine tasting, concerts, weddings, petting zoos, wagon rides, along with educational activities.

"The messages are still there about why agriculture is important, but it's in a more lighthearted way," she says. "Sustainable agriculture can bombard you with so many messages, and some of them are very dire and very serious. It's important, but sometimes people need a break from that.

"I think agritourism farms offer a great way for people to get out and enjoy a farm environment without becoming overloaded from the serious messages." Laughing, Mary says, "When they launch their pumpkin on the pumpkin cannon and it goes eight hundred feet, they're having a blast. But I hope they'll realize somewhere in there that they couldn't have a blast if that farm wasn't a part of their community."

Every October, Cascade Harvest Coalition farmers sponsor a Harvest Celebration. In between the corn maze, the pumpkin patch, and tractor rides, farmers talk with people about locally produced food and small-scale agriculture.

"When people go on farm tours, or they go out to the farm, I think they make that deeper connection. When they are actually on the land where their food is grown, people feel a greater spirituality about the food," Mary says. "People start to care where their food is coming from. And when you care where it's coming from, you also care about the environment, and the community, and the people. It completes that picture."

CASCADE HARVEST COALITION
4649 Sunnyside Avenue North, Room 123
Seattle, WA 98103
www.cascadeharvest.org

Then came *Silent Spring*. Rachel Carson had worked as a biologist with the U.S. Fish and Wildlife Service for seventeen years. Over the years, she had written a number of best-selling books that detailed the interdependencies of natural environments. One of Carson's hobbies was bird-watching. Over the years, she and her bird-watching friends had noticed the connections between wide-scale sprayings of DDT and flocks of dying birds or birds whose eggs never hatched. Carson found convincing evidence that when DDT was sprayed to kill insects, it then entered the food chain, accumulating in the fatty tissue of animals (including humans) and causing cancer, infertility, and permanent genetic damage. To make the public aware of the dangers of industrial chemicals, particularly DDT, she wrote her book *Silent Spring*, which was published in 1962.[4] The book immediately galvanized the American public.

I was not very old when *Silent Spring* was first published, but I can recall hearing my mother and her friends talking about how DDT was killing birds and fish, and the government wasn't doing anything to protect us. My mom had grown up in the 1950s believing, like many Americans, that the government would take care of its citizens and look out for their health and welfare. It came as a shock to her, and to most Americans, to realize that the government was allowing businesses to fill our water, land, and air with untested poisonous chemicals. For the first time in their lives, my family and many other Americans were talking about "ecology," "pesticides," and "the environment."

Carson's book was massively popular and very controversial. Chemical companies began a media blitz to discredit Carson and her book before it was even published. Many chemical manufacturers threatened to withhold advertising from newspapers and magazines that reviewed the book. Monsanto, a billon-dollar chemical manufacturer at that time, created and distributed a parody of *Silent Spring* to over 5,000 media outlets.[5] This parody, called *The Desolate Year*, told of a starving world overrun with insects. Monsanto and other pesticide manufacturers tried to use the controversy to spread their own message that pesticides were the only way to feed the world and control insects. This negative reaction by the chemical industry only gave the book higher sales.

The controversy became so contentious that President John F. Kennedy ordered the President's Science Advisory Committee to examine the book's claims about DDT. Although the committee concluded that pesticides were necessary to maintain the nation's food supply, their report completely vindicated Rachel Carson's research and her statements in *Silent Spring* about the dangers of DDT. Further, the report urged that restraint be used in the use of pesticides around homes and on food crops.

THE ENVIRONMENTAL ACTIVIST MOVEMENT BEGINS

This was the first huge environmental hazard panic to sweep across America, alarming the public and leaving the government rushing to try to do damage control. The amount of media coverage resulting from this debate created a new awareness among the American public.

Throughout the early 1960s Carson spoke publicly, encouraging legislators to regulate pesticide usage. Dozens of bills to control pesticide residue were introduced by Congress during the years following *Silent Spring*'s publication. The seeds of the American environmental activist movement had been planted.

In 1970 America's very first Earth Day celebration took place, with April 22 being declared by Congress "a national day to celebrate the earth." Schools, universities, and cities celebrated Earth Day with parades, music, and demonstrations advocating environmental reform. The Environmental Protection Agency (EPA) was also formed in 1970, with a mandate from President Richard Nixon to establish and enforce environmental protection standards, reduce pollution, and conduct research on environmental issues.

HIPPIE FARMERS
AND THE EARLY DAYS OF ORGANICS

Enthused by this new environmental awareness, some Americans began to "get back to the land" through farming, communes, and other collective living and farming arrangements. In Michigan, where I grew up, we called these people "hippies," and we sometimes wondered just what they were growing that made them seem so happy and mellow. The roadside signs outside of their small farms advertised "Organic Food for Sale."

"Organic" began to be used to define a way of growing food without pesticides or chemicals. However, the term was loosely defined and had no official standards attached to it. Consumers and farmers struggled with how to define organic food. If you stopped using chemicals, did that make your farm organic? Did organic also mean that your water source was free of pollution? What if you used pesticides one year but didn't use them the next year—was that crop then organic?

One of the first publicly accepted definitions of "organically grown" food was spoken in 1972 by J. I. Rodale's son, Robert, editor of *Organic Gardening and Farming* magazine, during his testimony at a public hearing in New York about organic foods. Rodale called organics: "Food grown without pesticides; grown without artificial fertilizers; grown in soil whose humus content is increased by the additions of organic matter, grown in soil whose mineral content is increased by the application of natural mineral fertilizers; [that] has not been treated with preservatives, hormones, or antibiotics."[6]

THE STATES TAKE CHARGE TO CERTIFY ORGANICS

In the early 1970s, after several years of functioning under informal organic standards, a few state-level organizations began to certify organic farmers. The Oregon legislature passed the nation's first organic labeling law in 1973.

The **California Certified Organic Farmers (CCOF)** organization also began in 1973, with a group of about fifty farmers who performed mutual oversight and certification of one another's farms to maintain agreed-upon organic standards. The organization quickly grew to encompass most of the state of California. By 1979 organic standards were state policy in California and Oregon, and were being considered in other states as well. There were still no national standards and no certainty that "organic" meant the same thing from state to state, or even locally, from one certifier to another.

By the 1980s the U.S. Congress decided that organic standards should be regulated to assure quality and prevent fraud. They began to try to establish national standards for organic produce, meat, and food products. The **Organic Foods Production Act (OFPA)** was part of the Farm Bill passed by Congress in 1990. The OFPA's purpose was to establish national standards for the production and handling of all foods carrying the "organic" label. The passage of the OFPA led to the creation of the **National Organic Standards Board (NOSB)**, which was charged with developing a set of standards for substances that could and could not be used in organic production. Thus the National Organic Program (NOP) standards were born.

As defined by the NOP, organic produce must be grown in soil that has been free of synthetic pesticides and fertilizers for at least three years. Farmers cannot use synthetically compounded fertilizer or fertilizer made with sewage sludge. Synthetic pesticides, livestock feed additives, bioengineering, and irradiation are also prohibited. Organic poultry, eggs, meats, and dairy products come from livestock that are given no antibiotics or growth hormones.

WHAT DOES IT MEAN TO BE CERTIFIED ORGANIC?

The difference between the earlier generation of organic farmers and organics today is that now farmers take products into the marketplace with a government-certified label to verify that their farming methods meet organic standards. The United States, Canada, the United Kingdom, and the European Union have organic standards to regulate the production, labeling, inspection and sale of organic products. Only growers who follow the standards and pass an inspection can sell organic products in those countries. Organic products imported from other countries are supposed to meet those same standards.

To become a certified organic grower in the United States, there are five steps that a farmer or food processor must follow.

1. **Find a certifier.** Organic certification agencies can be operated by a state agriculture department or they may be private agencies, but they operate as an extension of the U.S. government and must be accredited by the NOP. Fee structures vary according to agency

and range from a flat fee to a percentage of the farm's annual net income. Small farms generally pay a few hundred dollars for organic certification, while the biggest operations may pay as much as $150,000. In addition, organic certifying agencies charge a percentage fee based on gross annual organic sales.

2. **Obtain an application.** The certification agency provides a packet containing a detailed assessment that must be completed by the farmer. The grower must provide information about their plans for soil fertility, weed and pest management practices (including the materials they plan to use), plus storage and harvest practices. Farm maps are often required, along with three-year histories for all cropland. A strategy to prevent contamination and commingling with nonorganic products must be outlined. The assessment also requires the farmer's proposal to ensure compliance with their strategy plan.

3. **Finalize the application.** The certifier reviews the application and assists the farmer in working through any outstanding issues. The farmer pays the certifier a fee.

4. **Allow the farm to be inspected.** The certification agency assigns an organic inspector to make an on-site inspection of the farm—buildings, cropland, streams, equipment, and borders that abut nonorganic property. The inspector prepares a report for the farmer and the certification agency detailing the findings.

5. **Receive a final review and determination.** The inspection and other documents are reviewed by the certification agency, and a determination is made as to whether the farm should or should not be certified organic. If the farm is certified, the farmer or

producer may then use the "certified organic" label for their products.

Companies that handle or process organic food before it gets to your local supermarket or restaurant must be inspected and certified, too.

For more information, see the Certification section of the USDA's Web site (http://www.ams.usda.gov/nop/FactSheets/CertificationE.html).

In Canada, surprisingly, there are no legislative provisions that specifically regulate the production or sale of organic food. However, organic products are supposed to meet a comprehensive set of rules overseen by the Canadian General Standards Board. Compliance with these rules is voluntary, except in Quebec, where producers can be penalized with large fines if they are caught misrepresenting nonorganic products as organic.

WHAT THE "CERTIFIED ORGANIC" STICKER TELLS YOU

The "certified organic" label actually tells you more about what your food *doesn't* have—pesticides and synthetic chemicals, hormones, antibiotics, and genetic modifications—rather than what it does have. Doesn't it seem like the regulating system for food is completely backward in this way?

It seems more logical that instead of labeling organic food, conventional food should have to be labeled with the dozen or more chemicals used to grow, feed, store, and ship it out to market. That would present a more accurate and fair representation of the real reason why conventionally grown produce is produced and sold so cheaply.

While it used to also be true that organic food gave you an

assurance that your food offered wholesome nutrition, environmental stewardship, support for small farmers, and a smaller "footprint" on the earth, you can no longer automatically assume those benefits come with organic food. As large agribusinesses have taken over the organic marketplace in recent years, the scale of production has stepped up dramatically. The next chapter, "Organic Economics," addresses the striking changes in scope and in scale that are becoming increasingly controversial within the organic market segment. You'll also read about why many **ethical eaters** are now touting local, sustainable agriculture as the new golden child.

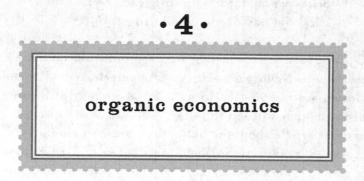

· 4 ·

organic economics

DID YOU buy something organic last year? What about last week? If so, you have plenty of company, both in North America and around the world.

* More than 66 percent of Americans bought at least one organic product last year, and more than 40 percent buy organics on a regular basis.[1]
* The global market for organic foods and beverages was valued at $23 billion (USD) in 2002, and was predicted to surpass $36.7 billion during 2006.[2] While the production of organic crops is increasing around the world, sales are concentrated in North America, Western Europe, and Japan.
* The United States demand for organic products is growing fast—demand was up 15 percent in 2005.[3]
* The demand for organic products in Canada has increased even more rapidly, going up at a rate of

20 percent each year since 1998. Similar growth
rates are also occurring in Europe and Japan.[4]
* The market for organic food within the United
States has doubled in just five years, racking up
sales of at least $14 billion during 2005.[5]

Organic food has reached the tipping point. The evidence is everywhere. Kellogg is making organic cereals. Wal-Mart and Costco are ramping up to double the amount of organic products they will sell this year. The *Wall Street Journal* runs another article about the business of organics almost every month. Ragu Organic Spaghetti Sauce appears on the daytime television game show *The Price Is Right*. The Food Network program *Unwrapped* recently aired a program called "Healthy Treats" that was entirely about organic processed foods.

BIG BUSINESS MOVES IN ON ORGANICS

The organic food industry has certainly become a victim of commercialization and profiteering. I had been buying organics on and off for more than twenty years, but after my daughter was born in 2001 I bought organics almost exclusively. That's a very common scenario—new parents start buying organics for their children, and soon the whole family is drinking organic milk and eating organic apples.

Now that organic food is the latest fad, nearly every food seems to be eventually reinvented as an organic product. If you haven't already seen them in your grocery store, you will—organic Dove chocolate bars, organic Del Monte tomato sauce, organic Frosted Mini-Wheats cereal, and many others.[6] Is that a good thing? Before I wrote this book, I thought it was a good thing. But what I've learned about organics as big business has changed my mind.

Just like every market trend, organics has passed through several stages of growth and has now reached the "me, too" phase—the point where everyone has jumped into the pool. The big food corporations have suddenly woken up and discovered that consumers are willing to pay more for food that is labeled organic. The opportunity to make higher profits is motivating them to reformat existing products as organic so they can charge a premium price.

SUPPLY PROBLEMS DRIVE PRICES UP

Although the popularity of organics within the food industry undoubtedly has had positive effects on farming, the pressure to find ways to produce enough organic food has also created a new and unforeseen set of problems. If you have been buying organic products on a regular basis, you may have noticed some evidence of the supply-and-demand pressures at your local store. During the summer of 2006 I went shopping at my local food co-op and noticed that for week after week the bulk bins of organic almonds were empty—no raw almonds, no tamari almonds, no grind-your-own almond butter. Finally, a sign was posted: "We cannot buy organic almonds at any price from sources within the U.S. We are researching the option of sourcing organic almonds from other countries. Stay tuned."

Hmmmm. That had never happened before. I found out that food producers who manufacture products like breakfast bars, cereals, and protein bars were buying up organic almonds as fast as they could. Bidding wars between companies quickly drove the prices up from around eight dollars a pound to fifteen. Small buyers like my food co-op were simply shut out of the market.

With the demand for organic foods doubling in just five years, supply problems are plaguing many stores that sell organics. While sales of organic milk increased 24 percent during 2005, the supply of organic milk increases an average of only 15 percent each year.[7] As a result, there was a shortage in organic milk supplies during the summer of 2005 (during hot weather, when the green grass dries up, grass-fed cows produce less milk). I have noticed that the price of organic milk keeps creeping upward at my local grocery store and food co-op, with prices now ranging from six to eight dollars for one gallon of organic milk at the time of publication (January 2007). Even organic apples were in short supply at times during 2005, as Wal-Mart began buying large quantities to stock their stores, and then other large grocers tried to lock up a supply of organic apples before they were all gone. The result seems to be not that organic prices are going *down,* as many predicted when Wal-Mart announced it would be selling organics, but exactly the opposite. Prices are going *up,* because the demand is high and the supply is lower than desired. According to an article in the *Wall Street Journal,* "Wal-Mart found the negotiating leverage it usually has with suppliers evaporated when it came to pricing organics because of the product's tight supplies and higher costs."[8]

Several mainstream grocers including the Kroger Company, Trader Joe's, Safeway, and Loblaws (Canada) have joined Whole Foods in selling their own organic branded foods, further straining supplies of organic ingredients. Raw ingredients, such as organic wheat, oats, corn, and almonds, along with out-of-season fruits and vegetables, are sometimes scarce as well.

Presently there are about ten thousand organic farms across America. During 2005, U.S. producers committed over 4 million acres of farmland to organic production (2.3 million acres of cropland and 1.7 million acres of range and pasture). While all fifty states now have certified organic cropland, California continues to lead the nation, with over 220,000 acres of certified organic farmland.[9]

While the number of organic farms in Canada declined slightly during 2005, the amount of organic acreage increased, as did the number of organic processors.

Many more farmers are aware of the benefits of converting their farm to organic production—lower input costs, profitable markets, and higher farm income—but their farm does not yet meet the requirement that cropland be free of synthetic chemicals for at least three years. This requirement is a significant barrier for many conventional farmers. Often farmers try to minimize the financial impact by converting only a few acres at a time to organic production. For example, they may have a five-hundred-acre conventional farm that has ten acres converted to grow organic tomatoes.

Another issue for certified-organic farmers is that they have supply problems of their own, seeing shortages of compost and manure for fertilizer or shortages of organic soybeans to use as livestock feed. These shortages drive up their production costs, thus making the idea of converting a farm to organics a bigger gamble.

Chinese Organics May Be Cheaper, but Are They Truly Organic?

Many of the big groceries and processors are adopting a new strategy to increase their organic supplies. In order to obtain large amounts of raw ingredients and cut costs, many food processors are importing organic crops from other countries, particularly China. During the winter months, I'm used to seeing anomalies like organic apples from New Zealand and organic cucumbers from Mexico at my local Seattle-area stores. Last winter, however, I suddenly started seeing organic produce from China. I wondered why organic food in the United States would be coming from China.

Here's the answer:

* The United States has 2.3 million acres of land for certified organic crops (the entire continent of North American lags behind every continent except Africa in total organic acreage).[10]
* China had 8.6 million acres of organic cropland (90% of its total) certified during 2004.[11]
* During 2005 China cleared another 7.6 million acres to be used for organic production.[12]

Curious about the mechanics of produce from China, I talked with Allen Zimmerman, produce buyer for the twelve-thousand-member Park Slope Food Co-op (PSFC) in Brooklyn, New York (see the profile on page 59). Zimmerman orders about 3 million pounds of vegetables and fruits for the PSFC every year, and has been doing so for the past eight years.

"The Chinese are major producers of so many organic commodities. They have so many climates, so much land, and, I'm afraid, so much cheap labor," he said. "The major buyers in the United States, like Wal-Mart and Whole Foods, are buying a good deal of Chinese produce. Not always as fresh produce, but often as the ingredients for frozen entrées or prepared foods. China is a cheaper source."

Zimmerman explained that there is no paper trail or way to verify the claims of organic certification from China—or from any other country's farms, for that matter. "I don't know how anyone could know," he said. "People who are more skeptical than I am may find it hard to believe that China is truly organic. This is a brand-new part of my world."[13]

Just as they have supplied the United States with cheap plastic trinkets, China is now poised to supply our food processors and the giant grocery stores with cheap organics. That seems odd to me, as China is known to have many pollution issues. Fred Gale, a senior economist with the USDA, has researched Chinese agriculture and told the *Dallas Morning News* that it is "almost impossible to grow truly organic food in China. The water everywhere is polluted, and the soil is contaminated from industry and mining, and the air is bad."[14]

WHEN EVALUATING ORGANICS, CONSIDER THE POINT OF ORIGIN

These supply issues are going to continue to arise for at least the next five years, and possibly beyond. Currently, about one-third of the organic produce sold in the United States is imported from Mexico, Australia, New Zealand, China, and Central and South America. Because the number of organic farms in the United States is increasing at a slower rate than in other countries, this trade gap is expected to grow if consumer demand for organic products continues to increase, as predicted, by about 15 to 20 percent every year.[15]

Amy Hepworth (see Hepworth Farms profile on page 28) made a special effort to call me after I interviewed her, because she wants you to know something. She says that farmers who are getting into organics now are only looking to make money. "I don't think they care at all about the environment," she said, "And I think people should realize that just because they buy organics, it does not mean they are doing something to make the earth a better place."

Buying organic food, even from far away, used to seem like the best way to increase the market demand for organics and to encourage more farmers to make that transition. Yet it now feels wrong to me to encourage shipping food around the globe, even if the food is organic, because it also encourages fuel consumption, paved roads, and polluted air. Just like the

EPA, I have to make a cost-benefit assessment, and I'm finding that locally grown food, preferably organic or sustainably grown food, feels like the better choice for me. Since I'm a math geek, I've even created a little formula that helps me to judge whether organic produce that travels a long distance is worth buying (see page 68).

I've noticed that many progressive food stores, especially food co-ops like the PSFC, where Zimmerman is the produce buyer, and the PCC (Puget Consumers Co-op), where I shop, make a point of letting customers know where their produce originated. Small Potatoes delivery service (Vancouver, BC, and northwestern Washington) also lists the point of origin for produce on their Web site, along with links to a profile of the farmer. I appreciate that information, and I do use it in my decision making. But stores like Wal-Mart, Costco, Whole Foods, and other grocery stores may buy organic produce from China and you'll never know it.

THE BIG O:
ORGANICS AND BIG BUSINESS

Just ten years ago you could safely assume that organic food offered wholesome nutrition, a safer growing environment, and a smaller "footprint" upon the earth. Organic farming was also supposed to be sustainable—meaning that the practices of organic farming were intended to steward the land, the farm animals, and the environment. But when large corporations entered the organics market, they started modifying traditional organic practices to suit the needs of big business. That's one of the reasons why you may now see small farmers who call their farm "sustainable" instead of "organic." As often happens when a trend reaches the mass-market saturation point, the visionaries and the early adopters who first began growing and buying organics have moved on—to local, sustainable food and farming.

For uninformed consumers the differences between certified organic and sustainable products can be confusing. For example, Horizon Organics, owned by Dean Foods, has been caught raising many of its organic dairy cows with thousands of other cows in feedlots where the creatures have had little freedom to roam, eat grass, or even lie down.[16] Since the animals are fed organic grain and do not receive antibiotics, Horizon can still legally sell "certified organic" milk. Many scientists agree that milk from dairy cows that eat mostly grass is different from the milk of grain-fed cows—it tends to be higher in certain healthy fats.[17]

According to a 2006 article in the *Chicago Tribune*, "Said Robert Fry, who served as a contract veterinarian at [Horizon] for eight years before he was dismissed in February: 'They portray to their customers that they've got this happy cow out on grass, this pastoral, idyllic scene. And that's not the case. There's a bit of misrepresentation on their part to the consumer.'"

Clearly, there is a huge difference between confinement dairies and sustainable dairy farms that strictly follow sustainable ideals, raise cows in a pasture setting, and produce high-quality milk. Yet, according to the government standards, the "certified organic" milk label applies equally to both producers.

GRADE B ORGANICS MEET MINIMUM STANDARDS

I care about organic standards, and I worry that these "Grade B" organic producers are continuing the same conventional farming policies that have created environmental and social problems in the past. The decline of small family farms, poor living and working conditions for farm laborers, a dependence on fossil fuels, and the breakdown of local economies in rural communities are among the problems caused by farming as big business.

Like me, many consumers who have been buying organic for years are unhappy that agribusinesses can deviate from humane livestock practices but nonetheless legally market their milk, chickens, or produce as certified organic. The organic label should mean something besides "this food meets the absolute minimum standards required by law."

Lucy Goodman, of Boulder Belt Eco-Farm (see profile on page 6) in Eaton, Ohio, talks with customers via her blog, through e-mail updates, and at the farmers' markets every week during growing season. She says, "I think that people are beginning to get it—that despite what our government tells us about us having the safest food system in the world, the government might be lying to us, and it's not that safe. Not only is it not safe, but the conventional food has no nutrition in it anymore."[18]

It's true that much of today's food is refined, colored, preserved, processed, and wrapped in plastic. Not because it is good for us, but because it is good for business.

Organics has evolved in just over twenty years to a product category that a majority of Americans have in their home. That change came about because people changed their purchasing habits and started asking for healthier choices. Clearly, we cannot just kick back with our organic TV dinner and let the food companies take over organic standards. It's important that you, the consumer, are well informed about food choices in your area; that you know how your food is grown; and that you have a store, a farmer, or a farmers' market that you trust.

Park Slope Food Co-op

As the produce buyer for the Park Slope Food Co-op in Brooklyn, New York, Allen Zimmerman orders about 3 million pounds of fresh fruits and vegetables every year. He purchases from local growers (the co-op defines "local" as a farm, ranch, or orchard within five hundred miles of New York City) as often as he can.

Allen is so passionate about supporting local farms that the co-op posts signs noting the point of origin for all of the produce it sells. During the summer and fall months, produce from New York State prevails. But during the late winter and spring months, produce comes from some surprising places.

A while back, the signs above the bins of fresh garlic noted that the co-op's organic garlic was grown in China. How did Chinese garlic find its way across an ocean and a continent to end up in the produce bins at a co-op in Brooklyn?

"Garlic is a good story," says Allen, who orders about sixteen thousand pounds of fresh garlic every year for the co-op. Finding enough garlic to maintain a constant year-round supply is a challenge.

"Most of the garlic in the United States, until recently, came from Gilroy, California," he explains. "But a few years ago, Gilroy's garlic crop pretty much failed. Because of over-farming in a monoculture, the garlic crop almost doesn't exist anymore. Even the largest garlic producer in Gilroy has had to import garlic from China for their packaged garlic products."

A little botany lesson is in order before Allen finishes his story. All garlic is botanically classified as Allium sativum, but there are two subspecies of garlic, the hard-necked and the soft-necked, with many cultivars of each. Hard-necked garlic is closest to the original, wild garlic. The garlic varietal that predominated in California, however, and now predominates in China, is soft-necked garlic. Soft-necked garlic was developed by growers seeking a garlic that was easier to plant and cultivate.

Now that you know that, let's get back to the story.

"Now the United States is importing most of its garlic from China, and China is dominating the world market," says Allen. "We, however, have now decided to get the best and most expensive garlic, and that is from New York State. This garlic from New York State is the hard-necked variety."

The hard-necked garlic that Allen buys for the co-op's customers must be planted by hand, clove by clove, with the root end pointing perfectly down. Hard-necked garlic also produces a flower stalk, which must be trimmed, again by hand, in order for the cloves to develop. "These stages of manual production make the garlic more expensive," Allen explains. "But it produces a juicy, powerful garlic. A memorable garlic—you know you've eaten garlic."

When New York garlic is not in season, which is most of the year, Allen tries to purchase his garlic domestically. "I try to buy as much California garlic as I can get my hands on," he says, "and when I can't get it, I'm buying Chinese garlic."

Shaking his head, Allen says, "It's a brand-new part of my

world. *The first time I saw Chinese [produce] it really shocked me. I couldn't see how it could make sense to get food from that far away.*"

Although meeting the demands of several thousand shoppers sometimes requires that he buy food from around the globe, Allen makes it very clear that produce from China is his last choice. "I buy locally grown produce almost to a fault," he says, "Yet I'm criticized for not buying more. Our members are more obsessed with supporting local farms than I am." Chuckling, he says, "That is because I am limited by reality, and they are not."

He strongly prefers to purchase food from the local farmers that he's come to know and trust during his tenure at the co-op. Relationships are very tight between Allen and some of his growers: "I give them my wish list and say, 'If you plant it, I will buy it.'" Other times local farmers will simply knock on the back door with a truckful of produce to see if the co-op is interested in buying. Some long-term relationships with farmers have been founded that way, and Allen is pleased to foster those connections to local farms.

He sees his job, that of supplying enough fruits and vegetables for twelve thousand New York residents, as a challenging puzzle. This month one "little local" farmer may be the only source for organic fingerling potatoes, and next month another farmer may have the only source for local radishes. "The more sources I have, the better variety and supply of product that I can get. Of course, the more suppliers that I have, the more relationships, the more juggling, and the more madness in my life."

Despite the juggling, despite the madness, Allen Zimmerman sees buying local produce as an excellent value for the co-op's customers. "The added value that our shoppers get from the co-op buying local produce is that they get vastly superior freshness and flavor. We've actually had basil harvested after sunset and delivered before sunrise the next day. In New York City you can't possibly get fresher."

PARK SLOPE FOOD CO-OP
782 Union Street
(between 6th and 7th Avenues in Park Slope)
Brooklyn, NY 11215

Buying Organic Boosts Local Economies

Although few of us can eat local foods exclusively, all of us can make more of an effort to purchase locally grown and raised foods as often as possible. Here's why it's worth the effort to seek out growers who live and farm in your community: *Buying local and supporting a local economy brings a wealth of benefits to the people who grow your food and the people who live nearby. When you buy food from people you know, you know their values, and you know if they seem genuine.*

I've said it before, but it's worth repeating: the "certified organic" sticker on your apple is just a substitute for firsthand knowledge of how your food was grown. Visiting your local farm and seeing the farming practices with your own eyes, or talking with growers at your local farmers' market, will give you more confidence than a certification sticker. When you can look your farmer in the eye and ask if she uses pesticides on her farm, or how she controls for bugs and weeds, you have a greater sense of control and trust with that grower.

Note to Self:
NEW WORLD ORDER STARTS HERE

The primary goal of many businesses is to make as much profit as possible. No smart person goes into business, including sustainable farming, planning to lose money, and I don't hold a grudge against any business for making a profit. To achieve profitability, businesses try to give their customers something they value.

What do you value? Cheap food? Americans may boast about having the cheapest food on the planet, but it's clear to me that we are paying the price in other ways—our health-care costs are skyrocketing from diseases related to producing and eating that food. My wife works in health care, and she sees so much cancer, heart disease, food allergies, diabetes, obesity, and chronic health problems—even in children. Many doctors and nutritionists would agree with her that these chronic diseases are often the price we pay for eating unhealthy food.

So, again, what do you value? I value whole foods that are grown in rich soil and that have taken in fresh air and clean water. I value food that is grown and raised by a farmer I trust—that is what I need to eat healthy and to be healthy. I believe that just like all creatures on earth, I instinctively know how to stay nourished, healthy, and alive.

If you agree, then you have to make conscious choices about food. Every time you make a purchase, you are telling businesses and farmers that you value that method of growing, harvesting, producing, and shipping that food. If you don't think big businesses care about how you spend your food dollars, think again. That's actually one of the *only* things they care about.

You have to take on the responsibility of making sure you eat healthy foods, live in a healthy community, and grow a local economy. No business, no matter how eco-positive its philosophy, can tackle that job better than you.

The greater value of building a good local economy, of shaping a community where you can trust your farmers not to pollute the air and streams, or to spray your food with pesticides, is that goodwill and trust becomes the norm. When you get to know the people who grow and harvest your food—when you hear their stories, when you talk with farmers about how and why they make decisions—you contribute to the work they do and help them contribute to a community of healthy people.

The next chapter, "Beyond Organics: Local and Sustainable," explores the newest trend in healthy, earth-friendly foods. Local and sustainably grown foods can be organic, too, but they provide additional positive benefits to you and your community. If you would like to move beyond shopping at the grocery store and get closer to the people who grow your food, the next chapter will explain your options.

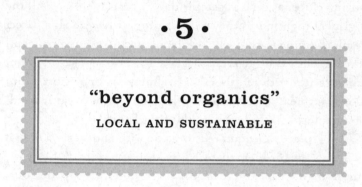

· 5 ·

"beyond organics"
LOCAL AND SUSTAINABLE

PEOPLE WHO have eaten organics for many years are now finding that the reasons they used to buy organic—to support small farms, to invest in the local economy, and to improve the environment—are no longer supported by the rapid growth in the organics market.

Many former organic farmers are now touting "buy local" or "buy sustainable" instead of "buy organic." What's going on here? Some organic farmers suspect that while they were busy tilling fields and turning compost, the food industry snuck up on them and took over the marketplace. Agribusinesses and large farms see opportunities to make money in the organic marketplace, but they often ignore traditional organic values like sustainability, environmental stewardship, and a connection to the local economy.

Virginia farmer Joel Salatin blogged about this phenomena in May 2005 after attending a meeting of large egg producers who were trying to find a way to fill the shelves at Wal-Mart with "cage-free" eggs. "I got the distinct feeling that the parties at this table on this day were far more interested in transporting cage-free eggs across five states to a Wal-Mart than in emptying Wal-Mart as a model and filling local CSAs, farmers' markets, buying clubs, and farm gates with . . . customers . . . All the logistical nightmares they were dealing with were all a direct result of trying to deal with a supercenter marketing concept, which I reject as fundamentally flawed . . . We replace one giant corporation with another."[1] (For more information about CSAs, farmers' markets, and other sources of organic food, see chapter 8, "Where to Find Healthy Food.")

"We replace one giant corporation with another." There it is. That's the problem many **ethical eaters** have with the growing demand for organics. Small farmers are opting out, because organics as big business is not how they want to farm. Most small farmers never dreamed that organic mac-and-cheese or organic TV dinners would have such a strong market presence, or that big-business agriculture methods would be associated with organics. Although their crops still meet organic standards, many former organic farmers have voluntarily decertified their farms.

When I shopped for organics, I used to assume that every company with a "certified organic" label followed the same standards, but I now know that different businesses interpret the rules differently (see **The Big O: Organics and Big Business** on page 56). Some organic growers hold rigidly to the traditional organic principles of minimizing pollution, eliminating chemically intensive farming, and humane treatment of livestock, whereas other growers meet the bare-minimum standards required to slap on a "certified organic" sticker.

Many consumers are beginning to understand that some foods are *more organic* than others, and they are beginning to follow the lead of the farmers by opting out of the current system and seeking alternatives to big-business organics. This has been referred to as the "beyond organic" movement. These organic alternatives are sustainable farming, locally grown foods, transitional organic, and Fair Trade.

SUSTAINABLE FARMING MEANS BALANCE

Sustainable agriculture is organic food with attitude. The primary difference between sustainable and organic farming is that sustainable farmers do not subscribe to a USDA certification process. Rather than following a strict set of laws or regulations, they incorporate ways of farming that will not deplete or permanently damage their resources and will thus *sustain* them.

The guiding philosophy of sustainable farming is balance—balancing the needs of the land, the community, and the farmer—to create a viable, healthy ecosystem. Sustainable farmers view the farm as part of a biological system and not as a cog in an industrial process.

Biodiversity and animal welfare are central tenets on sustainable farms. The farms raise a mixture of plants and animals that are rotated between several fields, enriching the soil and helping to prevent disease and minimize insects. Animals are encouraged to act upon their natural behaviors, such as grazing, rooting, or pecking, and they eat a diet that is appropriate for their species.

Farmworkers on a sustainable farm are paid at least minimum wages, and they are offered clean, safe living conditions and food.

Most sustainable farmers also try to support their local communities by banking locally, marketing to local restaurants and grocers, and supporting local food banks. Many sustainable farms do not use any form of chemicals. Often they were certified organic in the past but decided to let their certification lapse because of the cost, paperwork requirements, or differences in philosophy with government standards.

The Challenge of Focusing on Locally Grown Foods

Locally grown food is typically described as food that is grown within a one-hundred-mile radius of your home. Buying locally grown products from farmers you trust, even if they are not certified organic, can be a very good option if it's available to you. Buying your food directly from a farm or farmers' market will always give you fresher food compared to produce that's traveled thousands of miles to the grocery store.

An often-quoted statistic is that the average item in a grocery store has traveled fifteen hundred miles to get into your shopping cart. Visualize all of the fuel that was consumed and all of the pollution that was generated to stock your grocery store with its wide variety of products. It's enough to make you lose your appetite.

However, eating locally grown food exclusively is nearly impossible. Draw a circle around a map of your city that extends for one hundred miles in each direction, and try to eat only foods grown within that radius. It's difficult to do this in most areas of the country, even in the summer. In my region, I would only be able to find salad greens, a variety of seasonal vegetables, and chicken or beef. No pasta. No coffee or tea. No chocolate-chip cookies. Even basics like cornmeal and salt and pepper are not an option for most of us to buy locally. Trying to eat only locally grown foods is a noble goal, but it quickly demonstrates our huge dependence on fossil fuel to transport our food supply.

TRANSITIONAL ORGANICS:
MOVING IN A HEALTHY DIRECTION

In order to be certified organic, farmland must be chemical-free for three years. The term **"transitional organic"** can be used to signify that a farmer is using organic methods but hasn't reached the three-year requirement. Producing food without pesticides requires knowledge and good farming skills. It often takes at least two to three years before an ecosystem adjusts to organic farming methods. Managing pests and soil fertility during the conversion period can be a huge challenge.

During the conversion period, farmers have the disadvantage of not being allowed to use any pesticides or chemical fertilizers. At the same time, they do not yet have the economic advantage of selling their product as organic. Some stores and farmers' markets allow farmers to sell their product as "transitional" so that they can make money during the conversion period.

A "transitional organic" label is not allowed under present NOP rules. Some organic advocates support the "transitional organic" label, saying it can help farmers make the switch to organic methods. (Transitional produce is typically priced lower than organic food.) Although this is true, the added confusion of another organic label, and the temptation to big producers to use that as a vehicle to weaken standards, gives me reservations.

Transitional farmers do sell produce at my farmers' market and food co-op, and if the food is something (like apples) that does not grow in the ground, or close to the ground, I try to support their efforts.

Equal Exchange and Fair Trade

Imported foods such as coffee, chocolate, tea, vanilla, and bananas are sometimes labeled as **Fair Trade Certified**. These foods are often imported from countries where average wages can be as low as one dollar per day and living conditions are poor. The Fair Trade certification process began as a way to ensure that farmers and pickers reap social and economic benefits from their products. Just after World War II, Alternative Trade Organizations (ATO) were formed to improve living conditions and empower farmers in third-world countries. Most ATOs began as political or religious organizations to promote social justice and the elimination of poverty in third-world countries. Before the ATOs became involved, many farmers growing foods like coffee, tea, chocolate, or vanilla beans received only a tiny percentage of the supermarket price.

The farmers had been depending on middlemen and brokers to move their products through the supply chain to reach supermarkets in the United States and other industrialized nations. The brokers and middlemen kept large portions of the profit, leaving little for the farmers.

By working directly with local export-import companies, the ATOs were able to pay the farmers substantially more, and still offer competitively priced products to consumers. The ATOs also used their marketing power to make consumers (coffee buyers were an early target) more aware of the culture, educational needs, and living conditions of farmers and their families.

Later, umbrella organizations such as the International Federation of Alternative Trade were formed to reach a wider audience for Fair Trade products. Soon, Fair Trade certification organizations such as TransFair USA and others created uniform Fair Trade standards and labels. Once labeling standards were in place in the late 1980s, Fair Trade products really began to take off. This allowed products from around the globe to be certified as fairly traded.

Ultimately, these organizations came together and formed Fairtrade Labeling Organizations International (FLO), a unified global labeling organization. FLO created an International Fairtrade Certification Mark during 2002. Many imported products now carry the Fairtrade Certification Mark, including coffee, tea, rice, bananas, cocoa, sugar, tropical nuts, and spices.

When you choose Fair Trade products, it benefits farmers by eliminating the middleman and making sure that farmers receive the bulk of the profit from their crops. Often there are benefits for the greater community as well, such as schools, electricity, running water, or community centers.

Fair Trade Certified products typically cost about the same as products that are not certified, so buying these products is an easy way to economically support the farmers who produce your food.

FARM SUBSIDIES:
PICK YOUR POISON

Although it is true that organic, sustainable, and Fair Trade products can be more expensive than conventionally grown foods, you should also be aware that you pay a premium on food that is raised conventionally—even if you don't see that little detail on your grocery store receipt.

Congress passes a farm bill just before each presidential election cycle, which the *Economist* magazine calls "a gargantuan, five-year giveaway to America's farmers."[1] As of December 2006, the federal government had spent more than $21 billion in tax dollars paying subsidies to farmers (during 2006),[2] and billions more on subsidizing water and power suppliers in rural areas.

Here's how **farm subsidies** are distributed:

* Farm subsidy eligibility is determined primarily by the crop a farmer grows, not by his or her income level or financial need. Farmers who grow wheat, corn, rice, soybeans, and cotton receive more over 90 percent of farm subsidy payments each year.
* The vast majority of farm subsidy payments go to less than 30 percent of U.S. farmers and over half of these subsidies go to large commercial farms.[3]
* Family farmers with few acres who grow most of the four hundred domestic crops other than wheat, corn, rice, soybeans, and cotton received less than 10 percent of all farm subsidy payments during 2006.
* Farm subsidies are commonly known as the largest corporate welfare program in the United States, and you pay for them through your federal taxes.

It's as if only the kids from the richest families with the biggest houses could be awarded scholarships to college. In its present form, the farm subsidy plan just seems to defy logical thinking, especially because organic and sustainable farmers receive *none* of this money.

Instead of spending federal dollars for research on controlling pest outbreaks without chemicals, developing renewable fuel sources, or gaining access to new markets, the government pays conventional farmers subsidies to grow corn, wheat, rice, cotton, and soybeans. These farmers use plenty of chemicals, irrigated water, and fossil fuel. Then the government gives U.S. farmers an unfair advantage by enabling them to artificially suppress the price of those commodities on the world market.

How does the government do that? Instead of giving you a complete refresher course on macroeconomics and farm subsidies, I'll use corn as an example of how farm subsidies in the United State suppress corn prices around the globe.

The government pays farmers subsidies to grow a crop, in this example, corn. The subsidy pays for the "inputs"—seed corn, irrigation, pesticides, fertilizer, and other expenses—of the corn farmer. Since the farmers don't have to be concerned about the cost of inputs, they can use lots of water and fertilizer to grow tons of corn. They grow so much—tons more corn than they could ever sell—that they create a surplus of corn.

In other words, the supply of corn is much greater than the consumer demand for corn. As we know from economics class, when supply is high and demand is low, prices go down.

The farmers then store huge warehouses of dried corn, again with help from government subsidies. This creates a surplus of corn available on the world market. Because of the surplus, corn producers in other countries (who do not receive subsidies and must pay for their inputs) cannot sell their corn at a price that covers their expenses.

Government subsidies are one reason that free trade negations between the United States and other countries often become contentious. Many farmers in other countries feel that farm subsidies give U.S. farmers an unfair competitive advantage in the global economy.

Sea Breeze Farm

Sitting at his farmhouse table, looking out at the flock of brown hens strolling through the pasture, sustainable farmer George Page wonders out loud if it makes sense to keep chickens.

"We have a reputation for having some of the best eggs in the state. It's because we raise them in mobile huts, and we take the time to move them [through the pasture] every couple days, so they are always eating green grass. That is what makes the yolks so brilliantly orange," he says.

The huts resemble dome tents on wheels. Each hut provides a couple of dozen chickens space for roosting and egg laying, while the open sides let them roam the pasture. The chickens preen, cluck, and peck at grass as George watches them and wonders if he could ever charge people the actual price that it costs him to produce a dozen eggs.

"We move them, and feed them, and water them. We gather the eggs several times a day and make sure they are impeccably fresh," he says. "I know all of the details that go into producing eggs well. I know how to do it. But chickens are very labor-intensive to raise. Will people ever be willing to pay nine dollars for a dozen eggs? I've come to a point where I have to acknowledge that the chickens just may not be economically successful," George says quietly.

The irony is that chickens—or to be exact, a chicken—is what got him into farming. Living in the heart of Seattle with a degree in physics and a job at a start-up company, he didn't even think about farming. He did, however, think about food quite a lot. "Traveling in Europe, I encountered very high quality food, and I became interested in cheeses, French cheeses in particular," he recalls. "I was interested in having a goat or having access to fresh milk so I could try to make cheese."

Instead of a goat, his co-worker gave him a laying hen that he kept in the courtyard of his rented townhouse for a while. But when the building was sold to developers, George and his fiancée, Kristin, had six months to find a new place to live. "I would look at places in Seattle and think, 'I need a backyard where I can have a couple of chickens and a goat," he recalls, laughing. "But my [then-future] wife said, 'You can't have a goat in the city. It just doesn't make sense.'"

Finally, in 2000 they bought a farmhouse with four acres of pasture on Vashon Island, which is a rural island about five miles from Seattle. He bought twelve chicks and slowly began dabbling in raising animals and farming.

Now, six years later, Sea Breeze Farm has built a following among Seattle restaurants that feature the farm's products on their menu, as well as with islanders and urban dwellers who happily take a ferry ride and make the short drive to the farm. Those amazing eggs are definitely a draw, along with cow's milk, crème fraîche, heavy cream, and, yes, richly flavorful fresh and aged cheeses. Pork, beef, duck, and chicken are also available at the farm's store from time to time. The farm has recently begun growing grapevines, and their label, Sweetbread Cellars, is aging several barrels of red varietals that were produced during 2002.

Despite the farm's high-quality products, despite its devoted following, and despite all the early mornings and hard work, however, Sea Breeze Farm has yet to generate a profit. Many months the farm does not break even after expenses are tallied. That's why George is questioning whether it makes sense at all for the farm to continue to raise laying hens.

His problem is one of scale—his ten-acre farm is pretty small, as farms go. Farming on a rural island provides a mild climate, fresh air, and plenty of customers. Yet he's close enough to the big city that finding enough open pastureland to support the needs of his chickens, ducks, pigs, sheep, goats, and cows is difficult. In order to generate more income, George needs to either increase his production or increase his prices, and neither option is easy to do.

His dilemma is the same struggle that has led other farmers to use pesticides to increase crop yield or to use hormones to increase milk production. But George is not interested in going down that road, ever. "If I maintain my philosophies and my ideals about how I want to farm, there are some real limitations," he says. So he looks for other ways to trim expenses and generate revenue.

He reaches back to old-school farming traditions of frugality and eliminating waste to squeeze more value out of his farm and his products. He makes and sells chicken, beef, and veal stock, along with pâtés and sausages to sell at the farmers' market. If he has a surplus of eggs and cream, he might make a few quiches or fruit tarts to sell as well.

His love of cooking and his quest for better-quality raw ingredients were his motivation for starting to farm in the first place, so it's not surprising that baking offers another creative way for him to generate income. "I wanted eggs and I wanted cheese and meat; I wanted to make those for my own use. I was already making wine as a hobby. All the things that I wanted—those are the things that I grow now. I started raising pigs so I could make prosciutto and salami. I got cows so I could have butter and cream."

George Page says his customer base is so loyal and so knowledgeable about his growing practices and philosophy that there is no reason for him to become certified organic. "My customers are way beyond organics," he says with a shrug. "They want something better than organics. That's why they come here."

SEA BREEZE FARM
10730 SW 116th Street
Vashon Island, WA 98070
http://home.comcast.net/~georgepage2/Index.html
*The farm stand at Sea Breeze Farm is open from
6 A.M. to 9 P.M. every day. They also sell on Satur-
days at the Vashon Island farmers' market and on
Sundays at the West Seattle Farmers' Market.*

Making the Transition to
Healthier Eating Can Be Easy

You may want to make healthier choices, but it's hard to change the way you buy food. The supermarket is right on the way home from school or work, and it has most of the things you need stacked up and ready to take home. You never have to wonder if apples are in season or if tomatoes are ripe. Apples are always available at the supermarket (even if they've been in a temperature-controlled storage shed for eight months), and the tomatoes are *never* ripe. Low expectations, low quality, and low prices—all there for you at one convenient location.

The best way to make the transition from conventional foods to organics or sustainably grown food is to take small steps. Here are a few easy ways to start making that transition:

* If you've never bought organic foods before, try buying the Dirty Dozen fruits and vegetables organically or sustainably grown as often as possible (see chapter 6, "The Dirty Dozen: Twelve Foods to Eat Only if They're Organic").
* Pick the five foods your family eats the most often— say milk, chicken, apples, peanut butter, and lettuce—and try to buy them organically or locally.
* If your grocer doesn't carry organics, look for a food cooperative or a natural foods store.
* Look online to find farmers' markets, CSAs, or farm stands in your area and try to make a connection with a local farmer (see chapter 8, "Where to Find Healthy Food.")

When you go shopping at a food co-op or the farmers' market, try to go when you are relaxed and not in a hurry to get somewhere else. Take the time to talk with people—farmers, other customers, produce stockers, cashiers—and ask questions. If you see a type of produce you've never eaten before, don't just walk on by. Pick it up. Smell it. Ask the nearest person if they know what it's called or how they would cook it.

If you've been eating mostly organic food and you want to try buying local foods, try eating only local foods for one meal, or for one day. Find a farmers' market, or take a trip through farmland once a month to buy from farm stands. Some online grocery-delivery services list how far fruit and vegetables have traveled to arrive in your zip code.

ORGANIC OR NONORGANIC: A COST-BENEFIT EQUATION

When I was in my mid-thirties, I had an epiphany of sorts. After managing to avoid math my entire life, I learned that in order to pursue my business degree, I would be taking college classes in algebra, precalculus, all the way through calculus. As much as I loathed math, I wasn't willing to let it be a deal breaker for me, so I immersed myself in story problems, quadratic equations, and parabolas. If you have no idea what I'm talking about—well, that's the way I felt as I began Algebra 091, also known around campus as "Algebra for Dummies."

Fast-forward through a year of slogging through graphs and math problems. One afternoon I looked at a fence and realized that I could write an equation to express that shape. I looked up in the sky to see the trail of an airplane and knew I could write a function for that shape, too. Suddenly I had a new way of looking at the world. Everything could be explained with math. Once you begin seeing the world as a giant story problem, you can create an equation to express anything. (Well, you can if you have a lot of time to think about it and you're a geek.)

Here's the problem: during times that you cannot find locally grown foods, organic foods from far away may be preferable to conventionally grown food. It's unfortunate that we have to make that kind of trade-off, but sometimes we do. How can you figure out how to make those choices logically?

If you don't enjoy doing math problems as much as I do, you can use the Shopping Guide on pages 157—78 to make those decisions easier. But if you find math fun, read on.

I wrote this cost-benefit equation to give me a formula to know when it made sense to select local food:

$$B = (Q - 1/2 \ M) / t$$

Here's how it breaks down:

B = benefit,
Q = quality (on a scale of 1 to 1,000)
M = approximate miles product has traveled, and
t = time to obtain.

In other words, the benefit of buying a given food is equal to the quality of the food, minus 50 percent of the approximate miles it traveled, divided by the time (in minutes) it takes to obtain it.

Generally my quality scale is based on expected appearance and taste (for example, I know that strawberries in January will be awful before I take a single bite). An average piece of produce, in season, would be scored as 500. I automatically downgrade anything on the Dirty Dozen list to 100 points maximum. On the other end of the scale, a really fantastic peach from an organic or sustainable farm in late July could be scored at 1,000.

Are you with me? Here's an example. Should I buy organic lettuce shipped 801 miles from California at the nearby grocery store, or buy locally grown but conventional lettuce from the greengrocer that's located fifteen minutes farther away? Here's how they might compare:

California lettuce: $B = [600 - 1/2 \ (801)] \ / \ 30$, so $B = 6.65$
Greengrocer lettuce: $B = [300 - 1/2 \ (100)] \ / \ 45$, so $B = 5.5$

Therefore, the organic lettuce from California provides more benefit.

Let's try it again, this time with something a little more complicated. When I visit my local supermarket, should I buy conventional grapes grown in California or organic grapes from Argentina?

California grapes: $B = [500 - 1/2 \ (801)] \ / \ 30$, so $B = 3.31$
Argentina grapes: $B = [500 - 1/2 \ (7,000)] \ / \ 30$, so $B = -100$

In this example, I kept both the quality and my travel time equal, so the grapes from Argentina have a negative benefit—not worth it.

Feel free to adjust my equation to fit your own values when you are shopping.

The next chapter, "The Dirty Dozen: The Twelve Foods to Eat Only if They're Organic," explains why certain foods are consistently listed as the foods most likely to contain pesticide residues or residues that are over the tolerance levels.

· 6 ·

---

the dirty dozen

THE TWELVE FOODS TO EAT
ONLY IF THEY'RE ORGANIC

---

*I*T'S TOUGH enough just getting your family to eat fresh fruits and vegetables without adding the concern of pesticides to the list of things you have to think about when grocery shopping. Thinking about the possibility of dangerous chemicals on your food might even seem like one more thing to take the enjoyment out of shopping.

Relax—there is an easy way to minimize your potential exposure to pesticides, even if you don't always choose organic produce. You can significantly cut your exposure simply by switching to organic for just a handful of fruits and vegetables. Fruits and vegetables on this Dirty Dozen list should *always* be purchased from certified organic growers or sustainable growers that you know do not use pesticides. So many toxic chemicals are used in the growth and life cycle of these twelve foods that buying them organic can cut your pesticide exposure by 50 percent![1]

Washing a food does not change its ranking on this list. Washing or rinsing food may remove dirt, bacteria, and insects from your food, but it does not remove much, if any, pesticide residue. That is because many pesticides are taken up internally into the fruit, and residues are found all the way through to the core. Other pesticides are created to bond with the surface of the food and will not wash off. Peeling fruit and vegetables reduces some exposure, but it does not eliminate pesticides.

How the USDA Tests Foods
for Pesticide Residues

The USDA's **Pesticide Data Program (PDP)** tests for pesticide residues in food and animal feed by **sampling**. In a process developed by the **National Agricultural Statistics Service (NASS)**, random samples of food are collected and tested for pesticides and other contaminants. The PDP sampling program focuses its testing on fruits and vegetables that have been identified by the EPA as having set pesticide tolerances. The foods used for sampling are a very small percentage of the total food produced each year, but they are intended to represent fresh foods that are commonly available to an American consumer.

Prior to testing for pesticides, the foods are prepared as if they were going to be eaten—pears and apples are washed and cored, bananas are peeled, nuts are shelled. Note that as mentioned above, while washing fresh produce may reduce some pesticide residues, it does not completely get rid of pesticides.

The FDA enforces pesticide tolerances for all domestically produced food and imported foods (except for meat, poultry, and eggs, which are enforced by USDA) and releases the results of pesticide residue testing.

Since 1987 the FDA has released the results of pesticide residue tests on more than one hundred thousand samples of domestic and imported fruit and vegetables. Based on these FDA tests, the **Environmental Working Group (EWG)**, a Washington, D.C.–based activist group (see Resources), developed its Dirty Dozen list.[2] This well-respected roster was created from analyzing data published by the government about the most commonly consumed fruits and vegetables. While I value the EWG Dirty Dozen list, it was only a starting point for my own research, and therefore, my recommendations are not identical to the EWG list. Also, the information provided in this chapter about growing practices and pesticides used comes from many sources, and does not come from the EWG. I am the kind of person who is always very curious about "why." I spent a lot of time investigating and educating myself about why certain vegetables and fruits seem to have such a heavy chemical load and why others do not. I've talked with farmers, researched agricultural Web sites, reviewed university resources, slogged through government reports, and looked to other sources for the information about the foods on the list (as well as the foods in chapter 7, "To Buy or Not to Buy Organic"). Whenever I found information a Web site, I always double-checked it with an authority—be that a farmer, a report, or another resource.

The Dirty Dozen—or as I call them, the Twelve Foods to Eat Only if They're Organic—(ranked by how likely they are to contain pesticide residue after harvest) are:

1. Strawberries

Some organic growers joke that conventionally grown strawberries are so full of chemicals, you could grind them up and use them as a pesticide. But pesticides are no laughing matter. Sixty-five different pesticides, fungicides, and herbicides are registered for use on strawberries.

Strawberries are the most chemically intensive crop in California. Most commercial strawberry growers use methyl bromide, a toxic, ozone-depleting chemical, to eradicate all fungus, **nematodes**, microorganisms, and weeds, effectively killing every living thing in the soil where strawberry plants are grown. For the remaining growth cycle, the berry plants are drip-fed chemical fertilizers. Because methyl bromide can cause poisoning, neurological damage, and reproductive harm, the EPA classifies it as a **Toxicity Category I compound**, which is a classification reserved for the most deadly substances it regulates.

Nonorganic strawberries are highly likely to contain pesticide residue after harvest. When the PDP releases its annual list of produce samples with residues that exceed tolerance levels, strawberries appear more often than any another fruit or vegetable.

2. Red and Green Bell Peppers

More than fifty chemicals, including ten different organophosphates, are approved for use on bell pepper crops in the United States. Bell peppers are typically treated with insecticides two to six times during their growth cycle, as well as sprayed with herbicides, fungicides, **fumigants**, **nematicides,** and **algaecides**. Conventional bell pepper growers often fumigate their fields with methyl bromide before planting to kill weeds and insects. Peppers may also get a dose of Gramoxone Extra (a brand of paraquat), a restricted-use pesticide that has greater acute toxicity to animals than most other herbicides.

3. Spinach

Spinach is relatively simple to grow when the right conditions are present—sandy soil; a long, cool growing season; and adequate water. When conditions are not right, spinach is susceptible to aphid infestation, insect damage, and mildew. Because spinach is often grown in less than ideal conditions, conventional farmers use significant amounts of pesticides, fungicides, and herbicides. More than 60 percent of the nonorganic spinach tested by the FDA contains pesticide residue, including DDT, permethrin, and other highly toxic pesticides. Several organophosphates are used on spinach crops, including chlorothalonil, a probable human carcinogen.

4. Cherries

Cherries, like most stone fruits, are attractive to many insect pests. Aphids, eriophyid mites, tent caterpillars, webworms, and Western cherry fruit flies are the major invaders that cherry producers try to fend off with pesticides. Cherries are also susceptible to many viruses and fungal diseases. In order to bring bug- and disease-free cherries to market, many cherry growers spray orchards with a series of pesticides and horticultural oils beginning in the dormant stage in early March and continuing until harvest in June or July. As a result, tests of domestic cherries show the presence of more than twenty different pesticide residues.

Organic growers are prohibited from spraying trees with any petroleum- or synthetic-based pesticide, so they have to make a truce with the wild birds that eat insects that plague cherry trees but often consume the cherries, too. Organic cherry orchardist Lise Rousseau of Bigfork, Montana, said, "It's not impossible to grow an organic cherry, but it does take a little more effort." Rousseau believes that maintaining a healthy tree that can fight off viruses and pests, is the best way to grow organic cherries.

5. Peaches

Like cherries, peaches attract many insects, fungi, and diseases. They are typically sprayed with assorted pesticides and fungicides on a weekly basis from their dormant stage in March until harvest in July or August. The peach tree borer, a persistent and destructive pest, is often eradicated with endosulfan, a highly toxic pesticide with xenoestrogenic properties (see page 17).

6. Nectarines

Nectarines, like cherries and peaches, are a magnet for insects and diseases. Something about the sweet juicy flesh of stone fruits attracts bugs like, well, flies to honey. The same routine for other stone fruits—spraying the trees for several months with various pesticides, fungicides, and petroleum-based horticultural oils—is followed for nectarine production.

7. Celery

The celery plant is essentially a water uptake mechanism, absorbing plenty of toxins from the soil and groundwater in the process. Nonorganic celery is a major potential source of exposure to organophosphates, including the probable human carcinogen chlorothalonil. In FDA tests celery is more likely than any other vegetable to contain pesticide residue—82 percent of the samples tested positive.

8. Apples

This all-American fruit is a polished beauty in the grocery store, but it takes a lot of bug spray, fungicide, and horticultural petroleum oil to keep apples so pretty and shiny. Apples are attractive to many kinds of moth larvae, aphids, leafhoppers, mites, and various other critters, and are often sprayed five to ten times during the growth cycle. Some apple varieties are also susceptible to apple scab disease, which leaves brown patches on the skin, and many other fungal diseases. As a result, more than forty pesticides, herbicides, and fungicides are approved for use on apples.

9. Pears

It's pretty clear that insects enjoy fruit just as much as humans do, and pears are no exception. Pear orchards are typically sprayed about nine times during the growth-to-harvest cycle to kill mites, moths, **scale,** fruitworms, and fruit flies. Fungicides, herbicides, and petroleum oils are also sprayed on pear orchards to control weeds and diseases. More than fifty chemicals, including several organophosphates, are approved for use on pear crops.

10. Grapes (specifically those imported from Chile)

Table grapes like to grow in just the right conditions—a dry, hot climate, with deep rich soil and plenty of groundwater. Humid conditions can lead to mildew and fungus, while cold temperatures can cause damage to grapevines. The fall and winter weather conditions in Chile are ideal for growing both wine and table grapes, but it's easy for aphids, nematodes, Mediterranean fruit flies, and other pests to hitchhike in on imported grapes. That's why the U.S. government requires that all grapes and stone fruits imported from Chile be fumigated with methyl bromide when they arrive at a U.S. port. Also used on strawberry crops, methyl bromide is classified as a Toxicity Category I compound. Under the **Clean Air Act** and the **Montreal Protocol,** two political initiatives designed to protect the environment, the production of methyl bromide, a known ozone-depleting chemical, was supposed to be phased out in January 2005. However, the EPA continues to make regular exemptions that accommodate agricultural users, because "there are no technically and economically feasible alternatives." More than 60 percent of imported raisins also tested positive for pesticide residues, whereas only 30 percent of domestic raisins had detectable residues.

11. Raspberries

Raspberries are delightful fresh off of the bush, soft and juicy. Those same qualities make raspberries highly perishable and very labor intensive to harvest. And the bugs love them—masses of hungry Japanese beetles, spider mites, aphids, and fruitworms eat the fruit, leaves, and even the woody canes. Raspberries prefer warm, dry days with cool nights, and cultivating them in undesirable climates can trigger mildew or fungus, causing the fruit to rot on the bush.

As a result of these challenges, commercial growers typically turn to several pesticides and fungicides to kill pests, as well as synthetic fertilizers to grow larger berries. Raspberry samples tested by the FDA have tested positive for residues of up to nine different pesticides. Considering that raspberries are a favorite finger food of many toddlers and small children, it makes sense to be cautious about selecting nonorganically grown raspberries.

12. Potatoes

Potato fields are sterilized before planting with a soil fumigant that kills all of the soil microbes and nematodes. When the potato "eyes" are planted, a systemic insecticide is sprayed over the fields to kill any bugs that may eat the sprouts. A month or so after that, the first herbicide is applied to kill any weeds hardy enough to grow. Because most of the soil nutrients have been eliminated, synthetic fertilizers are dribbled into the potato rows every week, like an IV drip of chemical nutrients. Midgrowth, many potato fields are sprayed yet again with the highly toxic organophosphate Monitor to kill aphids, potato beetles, and other insects. Finally, to control **blight** before harvest, potato plants receive successive sprayings of a fungicide containing **mefenoxam** and chlorothalonil, both acute toxins. Given this chemically intensive growth cycle, it's not surprising that a majority of potatoes, especially Russets, test positive for multiple pesticide residues.

> *Buying these twelve foods organically*
> *can reduce your exposure to pesticides by 50 percent.*

These are the twelve foods that have the highest pesticide residue after harvest, according to the FDA's monitoring program. However, a review of the FDA data shows that certain other vegetables are also likely to carry pesticide residues. Carrots and peanuts are known to absorb certain pesticides and heavy metals from soil. Greens such as kale, Napa cabbage, and mustard greens, along with most leaf lettuces, frequently have pesticide residues. Again, as I've already explained in chapter 2 (see page 23), you must always be especially choosy when shopping for fruits and vegetables for babies and small children, because their developing bodies are more sensitive to toxins.

THE CLEAN FIFTEEN

Some vegetables and fruits consistently test negative for pesticide residue almost all of the time. Sometimes it's just not profitable enough to use pesticides on the crop, or the plant has a natural bitter or unusual taste that makes it unappealing to crop-munching insects. In other cases, natural predators do the job for the farmer. In the case of some tropical fruits, they will only grow in the right climate and have developed a very thick skin that protects the fruit from heat and insect predators. The next chapter ("To Buy or Not to Buy Organic") gives detailed information about the growing practices and chemical use for all of the foods on the list of what I call the "Clean Fifteen."

Here is my own list, based on the same PDP samplings as the Dirty Dozen list. However, these rankings show you the fruits and vegetables that are the **least** likely to contain pesticide residue, even if they are not organically grown. The Clean Fifteen are the fruits and vegetables that had samples that showed little or no pesticide residues year after year.

You may notice that many of them have tough outer skins, making it difficult for insects to feed on them. Others have a strong flavor that is unappealing. I keep a worm bin on the side of my house, where the worms, pill bugs, fruit flies, and slugs process my food scraps into a rich, fluffy compost. I've noticed there are a few things that even the worms and bugs don't want to eat—broccoli stems, cabbage, onion skins, pea pods, watermelon rind. Many foods that the bugs clearly have no appetite for appear on this list. I'm sure that's no coincidence; if the bugs aren't interested, there's little motivation to spray pesticides.

1. Asparagus
2. Avocados
3. Bananas
4. Blueberries
5. Broccoli
6. Cabbage
7. Garlic
8. Kiwi
9. Mango
10. Onions
11. Papaya
12. Pineapple
13. Shelling peas
14. Sweet corn
15. Watermelon (domestically grown)

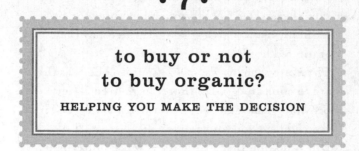

· 7 ·

to buy or not to buy organic?

HELPING YOU MAKE THE DECISION

*J*UST AS some humans adore the dry heat of the Southwest, some thrive in the cool drizzle of the Pacific Northwest, and still others enjoy the hot summers and cold winters of the East and Midwest, every fruit and vegetable has a climate where it grows best. Along with climate requirements, plants also have soil preferences, chemical sensitivities, insect appeal, and water requirements.

When a plant's needs are met, it's a happy plant that blossoms and grows. And when a plant's needs are not met, it will wither and die. That is Nature's plan for maintaining balance and allowing native plants to thrive. Cultivating food sources in disparate climates is not easy, and these plants often require special treatment to grow successfully.

This chapter details farming practices for many of the foods we eat. You'll also find the relevant factors to weigh when making the decision to buy organic or nonorganic when you shop as well as if it's best to choose foods that are locally grown. You'll also read some very surprising information about the food we eat.

* Why do some foods get so many pesticide applications while others do not?
* Why is grass-fed beef so much healthier for us (containing 50 percent less saturated fat) than grain-fed beef?
* There are as many ways to raise laying hens as there are to cook an egg. Do those "cage-free," "fertile" brown eggs have the edge over ordinary eggs? Find the right egg for your personality.
* Did you know that scientists now use butter pats from farms around the world to track the movement of persistent organic pollutants in the global environment? Read all about it in the Dairy section.
* Is it true that carrots are so efficient at absorbing heavy metals from the soil that they are sometimes planted to decontaminate fields that have been sprayed with sewage sludge? Surprisingly, yes, and you can get the details in the Vegetables section below.

FRUITS

Berries

Most berries are thin-skinned and grow close to the ground, both factors that make them pesticide sponges. Berries are also susceptible to mold and fungus, and nonorganic farmers typically use fungicides to give the berries a longer shelf life. Nonorganic strawberries are one of the most chemically intensive crops grown in the United States, and the extremely toxic pesticide methyl bromide is used on most conventionally grown strawberries (see page 85). Blueberries are typically low in insecticide residue.

Recommendation: Buy organic strawberries and raspberries—*always*. Berries are favorite finger foods for many small children, who can eat a box of berries in one sitting, so it's important to select organic berries for them.

If you go to a U-pick farm, you should always ask if they spray pesticides or fungicides before you pick and eat the farm's fruit.

Blueberries and blackberries tend to have fewer pesticide residues and are good choices for nonorganic berries. Berries freeze well, so buy organics in season and freeze them for eating in the winter months. Other berries are not widely tested for pesticides.

Stone Fruits

Because insects enjoy them as much as humans, nonorganic fresh peaches, apricots, nectarines, and sweet cherries are typically sprayed with several pesticides during the growing season. Cherries from the United States often have levels of pesticide residues that are at or above the EPA's tolerance levels.

Recommendation: Buy organic stone fruits whenever possible. Avoid conventionally grown peaches, as they often contain pesticide residues (see page 87). Canned peaches are notably lower in pesticide residues than are fresh peaches. There are three reasons for this difference: with canned peaches (a) the skin is removed; (b) the processing requires several vigorous washings; and (c) the varieties grown for canning require less pesticide to grow successfully.

If I am tempted to buy nonorganic cherries or peaches from the farmers market, I always ask the farmers how recently the cherries were sprayed with any chemical. ("Before the fruit set," which means before the fruit began to appear on the tree, is the answer you want to hear.) If any spraying has been done within the last month, take a pass, as appealing as the fruit may look, smell, and feel. Bottled or canned cherries can be an acceptable option (they test lower in pesticide residue for the same reasons that canned peaches do) if you cannot find organics.

Nectarines have high levels of pesticide residues, often from multiple insecticides. Conventionally grown nectarines should be avoided.

Of the stone fruits, plums have the lowest pesticide residue levels.

Apples and Pears

Apples and pears are consistently among the most contaminated fruits and vegetables. They are highly vulnerable to a number of insects and larvae that burrow into the fruit and destroy it. To fight these pests, the fruit is sprayed with insecticides several times during the growth season, and is often sprayed again after harvest with fungicides or petroleum sprays. Organic growers battle these pests by using sticky traps, enclosing the fruit in a breathable bag to keep insects out, or by sealing the apples in a cornstarch-based coating that repels pests. They also thin out bad apples by hand and destroy them.

Even after being washed, cored, and peeled, an average conventionally grown apple contains the residues from four to ten different pesticides known or suspected to cause nervous system damage, cancer, or hormone interference. Pesticides that are banned by the EPA because of their extreme toxicity, and some that are almost banned, are still found on apple samples.

Recommendation: Buy organic or minimally treated apples and pears. Organic apples, apple juice, and applesauce are found in most supermarkets and are highly recommended, especially for children. Organic apples and pears can be made into applesauce, juice, or pear and apple butters that can be frozen or canned for off-season eating. Apple juice and applesauce samples have less pesticide residue than fresh apples, but they do still have residues.

Citrus Fruits

Since orange and grapefruit peel are natural insect repellants, and orange oil is even used as a bug spray, you would think that oranges and other citrus fruit would be very low in pesticide residues. Alas, you would be wrong. Surprisingly, orange samples from conventional citrus groves often contain multiple pesticide, herbicide, and fungicide residues.

Citrus trees, especially orange trees, are vulnerable to many fungus diseases, nematodes, fruit flies, and other insect pests, and are sprayed with insecticides and fungicides up to ten times during the growth cycle.

Orange and grapefruit juices are lower in pesticide residue than the fruit samples, probably because they are vigorously washed and less fungicide is needed for fruits that are undergoing immediate processing.

Recommendation: If you choose nonorganic citrus fruits, avoid eating the peel, as that has a higher concentration of pesticide and fungicide residues. For baking or other purposes when you need citrus zest from the peel, it's best to choose organic fruit. If you do not have an organic fruit and you need to use the peel, one recommendation, from *American Pie* author Peter Reinhart, is to dip the fruit in boiling water for fifteen seconds to remove at least some of the pesticide residues.[1]

Tangerines and grapefruits present the lowest amount of residue for citrus fruits.

Baby Food and Kids' Juices

の

MANY STAPLES of a baby's diet are also foods that are highly likely to contain pesticide residues—peaches, apples, pears, carrots, green beans, and apricots.

A baby's growing body is very vulnerable to pesticides, even in trace amounts, and it is important to be very careful about any food your young child eats.

In just a few minutes you can cut up organic fruit or vegetables and simmer them in a little water. Mash them with a fork, puree them with a food processor, or run them through a food mill and feed them to Baby while they are fresh. If you make more than your baby can finish in one meal, freeze the extra in an empty ice-cube tray and save the cubes for another meal.

Nonorganic cereal grains, especially rice, often contain pesticide residue and should be avoided. A food grinder or cleaned electric coffee grinder can pulverize organic rice, oats, beans, or wheat into a cereal base you can simmer in water or milk to a smooth consistency for baby cereal. Many books are available that include recipes for making baby food. *Super Baby Food,* by Ruth Yaron, is one I have used, and it has recipes for easy-to-make foods that appeal to both babies and toddlers.[5]

Recommendation: Once your baby starts eating solid food, select organic fruits and vegetables as often as possible, and avoid exposing your child to the higher levels of pesticides, hormones, or antibiotics found in conventionally grown foods. If your day care or babysitter does not use organic milk and foods, take your own, and make them understand that your baby should only have snacks from home.

Commercially made organic baby foods, juices, and cereals are available in many supermarkets, but they may have added starches and preservatives. Look for products labeled "100% Organic," and read the labels to be sure that commercial products are not supplemented with artificial colors or flavorings.

Vine Fruits and Melons

Melons, such as watermelon and cantaloupe, require hot weather and lots of water to grow well. When weather conditions are less than ideal, the vines can wilt from mildew or fungus. When given the right conditions, their thick skins and wide prickly leaves are natural deterrents to many insect pests, although cucumber beetles, melon aphids, and squash vine borers can cause problems. Predatory insects are often effective against pests that are common to melons.

The majority of melons grown in the United States are not sprayed heavily with pesticides, because the vines are sensitive to chemicals (although herbicides are used early in the season), and they typically contain few pesticide residues.

Recommendation: It's okay to eat nonorganic melons in season. However, melons imported from Mexico, especially Mexican cantaloupes (which are typically sold in winter months), frequently test positive for pesticide residues and should be avoided.

Grapes and Raisins

Table grapes grown in the United States typically test low for pesticide residue. However, imported grapes test very high for pesticides (see page 89) and the highly toxic fungicide methyl bromide. Imported grapes, typically available during winter months, should be avoided, especially for children.

Recommendation: The best strategy is to buy organic when possible, or to buy only nonimported conventionally grown grapes from May through late September. Since they are a favorite snack of children, if you can't find organic raisins, buy domestically produced raisins. Domestic raisins tested positive for pesticide residues 30 percent of the time, whereas imported raisins were positive for residues 60 percent of the time.

Tropical Fruits

Tropical fruits such as bananas, pineapple, avocado, mango, and papaya are consistently among the nonorganic fruits least likely to contain pesticide residue. Specialty tropical crops such as soursop and sapote also test very low in pesticide residue.

There are two main reasons that tropical fruits have low pesticide residues. First, they are considered minor-use crops by the EPA, and therefore few pesticides or other chemicals are registered for these crops. In other words, there is not enough economic return to motivate chemical manufacturers to lobby the EPA to register pesticides for use on the crop. And if these crops are grown outside of the United States, pesticides are too expensive to apply as a preventive measure, so they are applied sparingly, if at all.

Recommendation: It's okay to buy nonorganic tropical fruits. Fair Trade bananas are a good option when you can find them. The Fair Trade sticker means the third-world farmers who grew the bananas were paid a living wage and their community receives some social benefits, such as clean water or health care.

VEGETABLES

Leafy vegetables

Most leafy vegetables are attractive to a number of leaf-munching bugs, slugs, snails, and other insects. Not only do the wrinkled leaves provide food, but they also make a great hiding place. Most shoppers don't want leaf vegetables with holes chewed through them. As a result, nearly all leafy vegetables—especially head lettuce, leaf lettuce, spinach, and mustard greens—receive at least one spray of pesticides during their short growing season. Among the pesticides commonly used on lettuce are the organophosphates Diazinon and endosulfan. Lettuce, spinach, and Swiss chard have also been shown to absorb toxic heavy metals when grown on soils that were sprayed with sewage sludge.

A majority of the nonorganic spinach tested by the FDA contains pesticide residue, including DDT, permethrin, and other highly toxic pesticides. Several organophosphates are used on spinach crops, including chlorothalonil, a probable human carcinogen.

Kale and collard greens are often found among the vegetables where samples test with pesticide residue levels in excess of the maximum tolerable amount.

Recommendation: Choose organic leafy vegetables whenever possible. Bagged organic salad greens and baby spinach are available year-round in many grocery stores.

Despite any inaccurate reports you may have heard, the 2006 spinach E.coli scare was not linked to organic products. The outbreak has been directly linked to four cattle feedlots adjacent to nonorganic spinach fields in California's Salinas Valley.[2]

If you are concerned about E.coli, organic salad greens *are* a safer choice than conventionally grown greens. USDA national organic standards require organic farmers to compost fertilizer at temperatures of at least 160 degrees, in order to kill harmful bacteria like E.coli. Organic farmers can only apply compost four months prior to planting.

On the other hand, conventional farms are not regulated in any way as to when they can apply manure to cropland, and the farmers are not required to destroy harmful bacteria before spreading compost. It is also legal for conventional farms to spray sewage sludge as fertilizer. Of course, this practice in banned on organic farms. Other greens are also best to buy organic and in season.

Underground Vegetables

Potatoes, carrots, radishes, and sweet potatoes all grow beneath the soil surface. With their thin skin and high water content, these vegetables all tend to absorb chemicals from the soil, even some pesticides that are now banned but remain in the ground.

Carrots are known to readily absorb chemicals from the soil, and they are sometimes planted as a throwaway crop to try to rid a field of heavy metals such as lead. Carrots planted in fields that have been sprayed with sewage sludge accumulate toxic metals or toxic **chlorinated hydrocarbons** from the soil.[3]

Sweet potatoes are typically lower in pesticide residue than are other vegetables that grow below ground, because many pests can be managed with predatory insects, and therefore **broad-spectrum insecticides,** or pesticides that kill many different insects, are not often sprayed on sweet potato crops. Farming practices, such as tilling the soil months before planting and rotating crops, are also known to be effective in reducing insect outbreaks on sweet potatoes.

Potatoes are grown in soil that is heavily fumigated to kill fungus and other diseases and pests. Multiple highly toxic pesticides, fungicides, and herbicides are sprayed on potato plants during their growth cycle.

Radishes have a very short growing season, typically less than thirty days, and most diseases and insects do not have enough time to gain a foothold before harvest. Radishes are even suggested as companion plants to repel pests in strawberry patches.

Beets for eating (as opposed to sugar beets) do not have a high pesticide load, although fields where beets are conventionally grown often receive a light herbicide spray when beet plants are small.

Recommendation: Buy only organic potatoes and carrots, especially for children. Be sure that potatoes and carrots come from certified organic farms that have been farmed organically for at least three years.

Nonorganic sweet potatoes and beets are an acceptable choice, as they are less likely to contain pesticide residues. Organic radishes are best, but nonorganic radishes are a good choice and have few pesticide residues.

Onions and Garlic

Onions have double protection against insect invaders—both the thick, papery skin and the pungent, sharp taste keep most bugs from attacking the bulbs. Onion maggots and onion thrips are the notable exceptions, and these pests are well controlled by crop rotation and natural predators. Thrips feed between the leaves or in the folded leaves of onion tops, making them difficult to reach with insecticides at all.

Garlic repels not only vampires, but most insects as well. The powerful antifungal compound **allicin** is released when garlic cloves are crushed or bitten into. Pests attacking garlic are likely to cause it to release this natural pesticide, and garlic is a well-known pest deterrent to interplant with other crops, such as lettuce and cabbage.

Green onions and leeks are sometimes sprayed with herbicide early in the growth cycle, because weeds compete with the plants for water and sunlight. Leeks have few insect pests and are not often sprayed with pesticides. Green onions may receive fertilizer to push them toward harvest sooner, but pests are easily controlled without pesticides.

Recommendation: Little, if any, pesticide is used on these crops, and usually no pesticide residue is found in onions or garlic. Nonorganic onions and garlic are fine choices. Organic green onions are often available at grocery stores and farmers' markets, so if you can find them, they are a slightly better choice than the conventional version. Leeks are acceptable to purchase nonorganic.

Cruciferous Vegetables

Brussels sprouts, cauliflower, cabbage, and broccoli are vegetables that typically have no or low amounts of pesticide residue after they are harvested. Hardy vegetables with thick stalks and tough outer leaves, they have some natural pest control. They are all vulnerable to aphids, cutworms, and diamondback moths (especially cabbage).

Broad-spectrum pesticides are not widely used for these crops, because the diamondback moth, the most prevalent pest, has repeatedly evolved pesticide resistance to almost everything. For almost forty years these moths have been sprayed with insecticides, but the moths become resistant and the pesticides no longer work. As a result, only mild insecticides are now sprayed, and growers have had to resort to biological controls that were pioneered by organic farmers, such as relying on the naturally occurring soil bacterium **Bacillus thuringiensis,** or **Bt,** and intercropping with plants such as mustard that are more attractive to the moths.

Recommendation: Nonorganic cruciferous vegetables are fine choices with low pesticide residues. Remove and discard the outer leaves of cabbages.

Green Beans and Dried Beans

Green beans are frequently found near the top of the EPA's list of foods that contain pesticide residues. Although they are not difficult to grow in the kitchen garden, cultivated beans are attractive to bean leaf beetles, potato leafhoppers, and European corn borers. Because all of these pests attack bean plants for two or more generations (as adults who lay eggs, then as larvae when the eggs hatch), several applications of preventive pesticides are applied to conventional bean crops. Herbicides are also commonly used, as are **mildecides** to control blight and gray mold. All of these chemicals add up to a significant chemical load when the beans are harvested.

There is little information available on dried beans from the FDA pesticide monitoring program, and dried beans are not listed in the products sampled by government testers. Pesticides and herbicides are used during the growth cycle of beans that are later dried, and some dried beans are fumigated while being held in warehouses before packaging.

Recommendation: Organic green beans are the best choice unless you know that your farmer does not spray pesticides or herbicides. Packaged dried beans may or may not have pesticide or fungicide residues, but there is no evidence either way.

Tomatoes

"There's only two things that money can't buy," songwriter Guy Clark says, "That's true love and homegrown tomatoes."[4] He's spot on—the best tomato is a juicy, vine-ripened tomato, preferably from your own garden.

Tomatoes grow best in hot, humid weather, and they are plagued by a multitude of pests and diseases. Many kinds of insects attack tomato plants and defoliate them or suck the life out of them, including Colorado potato beetles, thrips, weevils, aphids, and whiteflies. To combat the bugs, tomatoes are sprayed with several applications of different pesticides. Chemical fertilizers are dripped into the rows to increase the size of the fruit, but do nothing for the flavor of the tomato.

Recommendation: Even though tomatoes receive several pesticide applications, the majority of samples have few residues. When you can't grow your own, choose locally grown tomatoes in season.

Organic tomatoes do contain up to five times higher levels of the cancer-fighting carotenoid lycopene, the chemical that gives tomatoes their red color. Lycopene has been shown to have a preventive effect not only against prostate cancer, but also against breast, pancreatic, and intestinal cancers. At the grocery, choose organic ketchup and canned tomato products whenever possible for the additional lycopene benefits of organic tomatoes.

Cucumbers

Although cucumbers share many growth requirements and pest issues with tomatoes, the striped cucumber beetle is a widespread pest for cucumber plants. Since their sensitive vines wilt from most pesticides, only a few pesticides can eliminate the beetles without killing the plant. Unfortunately, malathion, one of the most toxic pesticides approved for use on food, is commonly used to eradicate these beetles. Malathion's known toxic effects include birth defects, cancer, chromosomal and hormone damage, brain and kidney damage, and childhood leukemia. Other organophosphate pesticides are also used on cucumber crops.

Recommendation: Nonorganic cucumbers are highly likely to contain pesticide residues and should always be avoided.

Winter Squash (including Pumpkins)

Pumpkins and winter squash are similar to melons in that when they have the proper growing conditions, few pesticides are required. They can be plagued by mildew if conditions are too moist or humid. The harvested squash are often coated with an "edible" wax coating to prevent mildew, retain moisture, and present a shiny appearance.

Recommendation: Organic unwaxed squash is better for food; nonorganic is fine for ornamental squashes and jack-o'-lanterns. If you buy nonorganic squash, avoid eating the skin.

MEATS

There are two ways to protect yourself against the harmful effects of hormones and other health concerns you may have about eating meat. One option is to consider alternatives to meat in your diet. A diet that is rich in many foods, especially vegetables, fruits, beans, and grains, is really the best option for everyday eating. When and if you do choose to eat meat, another helpful way to protect your health is to seek out good farmers and pay them a fair price for your meat.

As an occasional meat eater, I've decided that if I'm going to eat meat, it will be only from animals that are raised on a small farm and treated well during their lifetime. It doesn't have to be wild, or strictly organic, but the animal does have to be raised by a farmer I trust. Meat is not an essential food for me, so I don't mind seeking out good farmers and paying them for good-quality, humanely raised meat products. When you read the following accounts of commercial livestock practices in the United States, you'll understand why it's worth the extra dollar or two per pound to always buy organic meat or meat from sustainable farms.

Beef

Although federal laws prohibit humans, notably athletes, from using synthetic hormones to bulk up their muscles, administering drugs to dairy and beef cattle for the same purpose is a very common practice. Most nonorganic U.S. cattle are given muscle-building **androgens**—usually testosterone surrogates—to bulk them up so that they can put on weight before slaughter. Other cows receive estrogen, a female sex hormone, or progestin, a semi-androgen that shuts down estrus, to allow their bodies to build muscle mass for meat instead of deploying that energy to prepare the cow's body for reproduction.

Countries in the European Union, along with other countries, have banned U.S. beef that has been given hormones, because studies show that the hormones are a "complete carcinogen."[6] One 2003 study carried out for the Pentagon linked Zeranol, a synthetic estrogen widely used to fatten beef cattle, to an increase in the growth of cancer cells, particularly breast cancer. Researchers at Ohio State University mixed beef from Zeranol-treated cows with human breast cancer cells in a laboratory setting. The researchers saw "significant" cancer cell growth—even with Zeranol levels thirty times *lower* than the levels the EPA says is safe for humans. Concerned about possible long-term effects, the researchers wrote: "consumption of food . . . derived from . . . animals treated with Zeranol poses a potential health risk to consumers."[7]

QUICK AND DIRTY BEEF

Given all of these facts, it is shocking to me that a majority of the nonorganic cows raised in the United States for beef are still given synthetic growth hormones. Six **hormone growth promotants (HGPs)** are approved for beef cattle, and one additional hormone is approved to increase milk productivity in dairy cows. Hardly any other countries have approved the use of HGPs, and many countries have banned their use outright. But in the United States, where chemical manufacturers have well-connected lobbyists pushing their products, hormones are the quick and dirty way to fatten up cattle.

Remember how we were all terrified of mad cow disease in 2004? It was known as a time bomb in the human brain, slowly eating holes in the brains of people who had consumed meat from infected animals. Nowadays we rarely hear of it, mainly because the government finally mandated that beef producers stop feeding cows (a species that does not consume other animals and is not built to digest animal protein) grain that was supplemented with the politely phrased "animal by-products." In other words, until 1997 cows were given feed containing ground-up bones, blood, feces, feathers, and waste products from sheep, chickens, and even other cows. Feed manufacturers thought they could create cheaper cattle feed, as well as use up the piles of waste in a typical feedlot operation if they blended waste products into food for the cows. It is widely accepted that mad cow disease, or **bovine spongiform encephalopathy (BSE),** arose because of this unnatural practice.

Disturbingly, poultry manure (containing arsenic—see **Chicken,** page 112) and some animal waste products can still be added to feed for beef cattle. In January 2004 the FDA proposed banning the addition of poultry litter to nonorganic cattle feed; however, in October 2005, after taking comments from the cattle industry, the agency quietly backtracked and decided to continue to allow poultry litter in cattle feed. It's appalling that cows are still fed chicken droppings, but the "FDA has carefully analyzed the comments it received . . . and has concluded that the other feed control measures discussed . . . are not needed."[8] According to the Department of Animal Sciences at the University of Missouri, "Feeding poultry litter is a means of disposing of a waste product while concurrently supplying a low-cost protein feed to beef cattle."[9]

Exit Through the Rear

Cows evolved to eat only plants that grow in a grassy pasture—not chicken manure, not grain, not animal waste products. Because their bodies react violently to being fed a diet of grain instead of grass, cows receive doses of antibiotics when they begin a grain diet. Cows eating cattle feed instead of pasture grass become gassy, bloated, and sick to their stomachs. And, remember, they have seven stomachs. They are given antibiotics to lessen the effects that corn-based cattle feed has on an animal that was designed to eat only grass.

And then many of those residual antibiotics and hormones exit through the rear, ending up in huge **manure pools** that often overflow into the local streams, creeks, and rivers. Many studies have documented that fish and aquatic creatures living downstream from large cattle farms are very likely to have birth defects and deformations—many of them reproductive defects caused by the hormones. Birds and other animals that eat the fish and frogs near large cattle farms also show the sad effects of hormones in the food supply—laying fewer eggs than normal, or laying sterile eggs that never hatch.

Grass-fed and Grass-finished Beef

So what's a meat eater to do? If you want to continue to have beef in your diet, seek out a source for grass-fed or grass-finished organic beef. Organic beef means that no hormones or antibiotics were given to the cattle, that the cattle had access to the organic fields for grazing, and that any feed was organically produced and free of animal by-products.

Grass-fed cattle are free to graze on grasses, clover, alfalfa, and other greens throughout their life, which is the natural diet for a cow. Beef from grass-fed cattle has many health benefits over grain-fed beef.[10] Grass-fed beef has nearly six times more **omega-3 fatty acids** than the grain-fed beef that is typically found in grocery stores. In addition, grass-fed beef contains almost no omega-6—that's the saturated fat that clogs arteries. Meat from a typical grain-fed steer contains twice as much fat when compared to meat from a grass-fed steer.[11]

Stores such as Whole Foods, Wild Oats, and natural food cooperatives are potential sources of grass-fed beef, but finding a local rancher is your best option (see Resources to locate grass-fed beef in your area). Some producers will ship organic or grass-fed beef or other products to interested consumers. Niman Ranch, based in Marin County, California, ships sustainable farm-raised high-quality cuts of beef, pork, and lamb anywhere in the country. My daughter is a fan of their "Fearless Uncured Beef Franks," which are hot dogs made with only quality cuts of beef and pork, and cured without nitrites.

Be cautious about beef or any meat at the supermarket that is labeled "Natural" or "All Natural," as those labels have no definitive meaning. If you are in doubt, research the rancher or beef's producer before you purchase it. If you choose the cheapest nonorganic meats at your local supermarket, you're getting "more" for your money than you think.

Chicken

Commercial chicken raising is a relentless grind. Chickens that are raised for meat typically have about fifty days of life, and as with other farm animals raised for meat, the goal is to get them fattened up as quickly as possible. To this end, the chickens are typically raised with about twenty-five thousand other chickens in large sheltered warehouses under artificial light where there is little to do but eat. Within six to eight weeks they end up plucked and wrapped in plastic for display at the supermarket's "wall of chicken" (as my daughter calls it).

It seems hard to believe, but arsenic is a U.S. government–approved dietary supplement for animals and is found in many drugs added to poultry and other animal feeds. Roxarsone (4-hydroxy-3-nitrophenyl arsenic acid) is the most often used additive among the group of arsenic compounds added to the feed of broiler chickens to control certain types of intestinal parasites. Although there are many other sources of arsenic exposure for humans, including drinking water, seafood, and building materials, chicken can also contribute to arsenic levels in your body. Over 70 percent of the chickens raised commercially for meat in the United States are given arsenic in their chicken feed.

PLAYING CHICKEN

Chicken producers and feed supplement manufacturers like to claim that none of the arsenic in chicken feed is found in the meat. But the USDA's own scientists, writing in 2004 in *Environmental Health Perspectives,* a journal of the National Institute of Health, warned that arsenic levels in chicken meat are a lot higher than previously acknowledged.

The government's testing method involves testing only chicken livers (which metabolize toxins and are much higher in arsenic than meat), not the meat that most consumers actually eat. The Institute for Agriculture and Trade Policy decided to actually test chicken meat for arsenic levels in their 2006 study, *Playing Chicken: Avoiding Arsenic in Your Meat.* They tested chicken samples from supermarkets (both organic and nonorganic producers) and fast-food restaurants, and published the results, showing arsenic levels by brand name or restaurant name.

Almost three-quarters of conventional brands of chicken contained detectable levels of arsenic. Of the nonconventional brands (including halal and Amish chickens, along with organic and free-range chickens), only one-third had detectable arsenic levels. Although the arsenic levels varied among the fast-food chicken samples, all of the samples had detectable levels of arsenic.[13]

ARSENIC: DEADLY POISON OR CHICKEN FEED?

Conventional chicken producers claim that the arsenic in chicken feed is harmless to humans, another arcane chemistry-based argument, which is simply not true. Arsenic is a well-known toxic, cancer-causing, health destroying poison. New scientific evidence also shows that like many other agricultural chemicals, arsenic appears to be a potent endocrine disrupter at extremely low levels of exposure.[14]

And there's another problem with nonorganic chicken. The more than 8 billion chickens raised for food in America each year create a huge mountain of arsenic-tainted chicken po—, okay, let's call it manure. That's what they call it at the garden center after it's packaged up in plastic bags and sold as garden fertilizer. Pelleted chicken manure fertilizer for spreading around your vegetable garden provides yet another route for human exposure to arsenic.

Arsenic in animal feed is banned in the European Union and many other countries. Organic chickens are raised without arsenic-supplemented feed, without antibiotics, and without hormones. Especially if you have young children who eat chicken, or if you eat chicken frequently, it's important to try to choose your chicken wisely. Buy organic chicken, buy Rosie or Rocky Natural Chickens (the *Playing Chicken* study found the meat of these chickens did not contain arsenic; see Petaluma Poultry in Resources for more information on natural and organic chicken), or find a sustainable chicken farmer near you by searching the database at www.eatwellguide.org. Many grocery stores, such as Trader Joe's, Whole Foods, and Wild Oats, carry organic chicken meat, and most grocery stores can order it if customers request it.

Whistling Train Farm

Along a picturesque strip of land in Kent, Washington, in a pasture of green grass with a view of Mount Rainier, four lucky cows lay chewing their cud. Across the road, Violet, Edna, and Mrs. Fig (the Pig) root around in their pens snorting and grunting happily while their piglets munch from a trough of gourmet vegetable scraps delivered from one of Seattle's best restaurants.

Whistling Train Farm, run by Shelley Pasco and Mike Verdi, is an eighteen-acre farm where such leafy greens as lettuce, kale, Swiss chard, and collards grow in neat rows surrounded by tangles of wild blackberry bushes, chickweed, and other vegetation. A lot of farmers would call those extraneous plants "weeds," but to Shelley, who does not believe in using herbicides, they are just part of a natural habitat—for birds, predatory insects, and other creatures that she sees as a vital part of the farm's ecosystem.

Shelley feels strongly that farming without chemicals is the best way to farm, and to her, it's that simple. Case closed. She remembers a conversation with Mike when they first started farming about why she wouldn't use herbicides. Smiling, she recalls, "I finally said, 'Because that's just the way it's going to be, Honey.'"

Mike, on the other hand, comes from a conventional farming background where spraying herbicides to kill weeds was common practice. "I had a fifty-acre farm and two people," he says, recalling how he farmed thirty years ago. "I had five acres of carrots, and I could go out there and in a half hour kill all of the weeds. Now it takes us two weeks and five people," he says wryly. "It's hard to find five people, let alone five people who can do it right. And it's not just one time—as the carrots are growing, we have to weed them two or three different times."

"I've been watching my good friend down the road here, and it's kind of funny," Mike says. "He incorporates herbicides in his pumpkin patch. Now, that herbicide needs just the right amount of water. If you don't have that, you get spotty weeds. Now he's got a crew out there with hoes digging up the weeds. Lately it seems like he's using more and more crew. I've seen him do that with several different crops. But when I talk to him, he says, 'I don't know how you guys do it without any chemicals; I pour on the chemicals.'"

Some of his old farming buddies kid him about his new "organic" lifestyle, Mike says, but he is proud that Shelley has been so successful at growing food without using synthetic pesticides, herbicides, or fertilizers. "We don't have to market our ducks or our pork," he says, "because now people come to us. It's just word-of-mouth. They know we're clean, and they trust us."

"Everything about farming has changed so much in the last twenty years," says Shelley. "I've wanted to farm since I was ten, but when I was in my twenties and busy into my graphic arts career, I went on farm tours and started thinking about the possibilities. I realized that it was possible to do it the way I wanted."

Mike acknowledges that the transition from conventional farmer to sustainable farmer has not been easy for him. "It's been painful for me," he admits. "Basically, I call this Shelley's farm. She knows everything ever written in a book, she knows plants, she knows growing methods—she's got that kind of memory. She knows all of the different bugs, and she knows the good bugs from the bad bugs," he says with a chuckle. "To me, they're all just bugs."

Whistling Train Farm produces more than fifty vegetables throughout the year, including squash, cucumbers, beans, peas, and carrots. They sell produce and meat to two Seattle restaurants, and they have around one hundred CSA members who buy spring, summer, or winter shares. Twice a week they sell beautiful leafy greens, other vegetables, and eggs at two Seattle farmers' markets.

Shelley has a soft spot for farm animals, especially pigs, so in addition to about a dozen pigs, they also have a flock of two hundred chickens, forty fuzzy yellow ducklings, three cows and a bull, four cats, two dogs, and one bunny rabbit.

Shelley sells some of her pigs to other farmers, some to a Seattle restaurant, and some to her farmers market customers who want meat from a sustainable farm. They do use a worm medication for the pigs (see page 121), but otherwise the pigs enjoy a natural life, eating organic feed and munching organic vegetable scraps from the farm and one of the restaurants. Shelley and Mike used to sell pork at the farmers' markets, but they found it difficult to maintain a steady inventory, so they've changed their strategy.

Now a few customers who are willing to pony up the money ahead of time can "buy in" on a litter of pigs, purchasing either a whole or half pig. "It's basically like we're raising your pig," says Mike. After the piglets are born, the farm raises them for the customers until they reach slaughter weight. "If we do it that way," says Mike, "we can have [a local butcher] come out here and farm slaughter, take it to his shop, wrap it up, and you can take it home. We don't have to take the pigs to the slaughterhouse. It's kinder to the pigs and they are not stressed at all. Our guy never misses; I've never even heard a squeal."

Those four contented cows arrived one day after Shelley finally found her cow. "I first started talking to Mike about cow[s] shortly after we met," she says. "After I miscarried [before children Della and Cosmo were born], part of my therapy was to visit local dairies in search of a cow."

Mike knew that if Shelley was looking for a cow, she was going to bring one home. He figured he should get busy working on the fence around the pasture.

"I'm still putting up the fence when a trailer pulls up, and it's a huge trailer," recalls Mike. "First they pull out the Dexter, which is a half-sized cow. Then I turn around and they're taking a dog crate out of the trailer. I thought okay, I guess you have to have a baby to get milk, and sure enough, there was a little one."

Raising his eyebrows, he says, "Then I turned around again and there was another dog crate, so I thought, 'Well, we got two babies.' Then I turn around again, and out comes this almost full-size half-Dexter and half-Holstein cow. By then I said, 'Okay, Shelley, what's going on here?' and she said, 'Well, I got such a good deal that I couldn't resist.'" He rolls his eyes, but it's pretty easy to tell that he adores his wife, and that he's come to see the benefits of sustainable farming, Shelley style.

Licorice, Skunky, and the other two cows wander around the grassy pasture, listening to the trains roll by, stepping over the chickens pecking in the pasture, and eating all the grass they can hold. Shelley happily milks her cow, by hand, every morning and every evening (with a little help from the neighbor). Mike and Shelley have created a peaceful place together—a farm that sustains not only the animals, but also their children, their customers, their farmworkers, and their land.

WHISTLING TRAIN FARM
27112 78th Avenue South
Kent, WA 98032
www.whistlingtrainfarm.com

Pork

The story of commercially farmed pork in the United States doesn't have much happy news, either. Much of the pork produced in the United States is raised on very large factory farms where most aspects of the production (food, slaughter, processing) are controlled by a remote corporate office. The top seven pork producers control 75 percent of the market for pork. Pigs are treated as a commodity—literally. Pork belly futures are traded at the Chicago Mercantile Exchange.

As such, pigs are confined in small stackable pens like products in a warehouse and given vitamins, hormones, and antibiotics routinely. Their tails are chopped off to keep the bored and frustrated pigs from biting them off. Sows spend most of their life in metal crates with barely enough room to lie down and nurse their piglets without crushing them.

A Spray of Eau de Porcs

Giant "lagoons" of pig manure from huge factory farms stink up the surrounding areas and often overflow into the local creeks, rivers, and streams. The ultimate destination of this lake of pig waste, contaminated with antibiotics and hormones, is as crop fertilizer to nonorganic farms. Pig manure, untreated and unsanitized, is routinely sprayed over conventionally grown food crops that you eat.

Contrast that image with the way pigs are raised by Mike Verdi and Shelly Pasco at sustainable Whistling Train Farm in Kent, Washington (see page 115). "We treat our sows as humanely as we possibly can and raise the baby pigs in a stress-free environment. Our pigs are all given lots of room to exercise and fulfill their pig instincts. This means they can root around in the dirt, sleep in the sun, eat vegetation, and run and chase each other. This makes for happy, healthy pigs that rarely need any medication. We use an excellent-quality organic feed in addition to access to outdoor pasture and the farm's surplus produce."

Instead of trucking the pigs to a slaughter facility where they might wait for hours or even days listening to the squealing of other terrified pigs, Whistling Train Farm has a butcher who comes to the farm to do the job and prepare the meat. It's hard to know how the pigs feel about it, but given that we all have to go someday, if I were a pig, I'd want to live my life on a farm where they cared at least that much.

ORGANIC PIGS ARE RARE

Although factory farms are not good places to support with your dollars, organically grown pork can be difficult, but not impossible, to find. Pigs are tricky to raise organically for several reasons. Pigs cannot meet all of their nutritional needs from grazing or foraging as most other farm animals do. They need protein in their diet, which most often comes from soybeans, and sources for organic soybeans are limited.

Pigs, especially pigs that can roam and root outdoors (which is their natural behavior), are susceptible to roundworm parasites that affect their intestines, lungs, and liver. Pigs infested with parasites cannot absorb nutrients and become sickly, and such roundworm infestations can quickly spread to become an epidemic. With no organic treatments for roundworms, few pig farmers have the perfect conditions to successfully raise pigs organically. As a result, organic pork is difficult to find. The best strategy is to find a farmer in your area who will talk with you about their farming methods and will allow you to visit the farm so that you can see the conditions with your own eyes. If there are no sustainable or organic farms in your area that raise pigs, mail-order sources such as Niman Ranch or Diamond Organics (see Resources) can be good options.

Dairy Products

Milk

Organic milk is considered a "gateway" product for new organic consumers, meaning it is typically the first organic product purchased by shoppers who are new to organic products. Purchases of organic milk in the United States have gone up 126 percent since 2000.[15] I believe that a great deal of this increase is from parents who choose organic milk for their young children because of concerns over the **rBGH** and **rBST growth hormones** given to nonorganic dairy cows. With sales of $322 million in 2005,[16] organic milk has become such a market force that some nonorganic dairies are stopping their use of these unpopular hormones to try to gain back the market share lost to organic producers.

VEGANS HAVE FEWER TWINS THAN VEGETARIANS

There is good reason for parents to be choosing organic milk in record numbers. Recent studies suggest that the synthetic growth hormones used to increase milk production in nonorganic dairy cows may be carcinogenic. Scientists also think that exposure to these hormones in nonorganic milk can be linked to the preteen onset of puberty in girls.[17]

New research also shows a likely link between growth hormones in milk and increased twin rates. Although in vitro fertilization and women having children later in life both play into the increase in the rate of twins, the United Kingdom, where bovine growth hormones are banned, saw only a 16 percent increase in twins during 1992–2001, while the U.S. rate increased by 32 percent.

Physician Gary Steinman of the Long Island Jewish Medical Center blames growth hormones in milk for a portion of the rise in the incidence of twins in the United States. Steinman and his colleagues compared twin rates between omnivore/vegetarian women (whose diets may include eggs and dairy products) and vegan women (who consume no animal products at all). He found that the omnivore/vegetarian women were five times more likely to have fraternal twins. Steinman contends that "insulin-like growth factor," a protein released by a woman's liver in response to stimulation from bovine growth hormones, is the likely reason. Other studies back up his assertion that the presence of the protein in a woman's body increases ovulation. Drinking one glass of nonorganic milk a day over a twelve-week period increased levels of the protein in a woman's body by 10 percent. Vegan women were found to have 13 percent lower concentrations of "insulin-like growth factor" in their blood.[18]

Clearly, it's best to avoid milk with growth hormones. There is plenty of evidence that the hormones given to dairy cows are passed through to the milk they produce, and that those hormones can cause significant changes to the human body. Remember that even tiny, tiny amounts of hormones have an effect of the endocrine (hormone) system (see Chapter 2, Babies and Small Children May Be Exposed during Critical Developmental Periods, page 23). Choosing organic milk is the best way to avoid ingesting undesirable growth hormones through milk.

GOOD MILK, GOOD FUN

Many small dairies dot the rural countryside, where cows are raised on grassy pastures with plenty of fresh air and humane living conditions. These small dairies can provide you with the freshest, best-tasting milk you've ever had. At Sea Breeze Farm on Vashon Island, Washington, farmer George Page raises dairy cows, goats, chicken, ducks, and pigs on a wide patchwork of grassy fields (see the profile of Sea Breeze Farm on page 74). The lactating animals always have dibs on the best, grassiest fields for grazing—first the cows, then the goats.

When my daughter and I head over to the island to buy food from Sea Breeze Farm, we are greeted by a gang of friendly farm dogs, clucking chickens, and crowing roosters. Milk, eggs, cheese, and other foods are in the refrigerator in the farm's store, and customers help themselves, tallying up the total and leaving payment in a bucket. Everything is fresh, clean, neatly labeled, and delicious.

My daughter and I happened to end up there one afternoon at milking time, and she was absolutely mesmerized by the process. I've talked with George about his growing methods, I've toured his farm, and I've tasted the food he produces. It's obvious he loves the work he does, and it shows in everything he produces.

If you don't know of a small dairy in your area, the Organic Valley cooperative (see Resources) provides milk from small dairies to many groceries. The cooperative is a group of more than seven hundred small dairies that produce the Organic Valley family of organic milk, dairy products, butter, eggs, and cheese. The cooperative supplies marketing and distribution routes so that many small family dairies can stay in business.

Recommendation: Buy organic milk exclusively, especially for children, unless you can go to a small dairy that raises dairy cows in a sustainable way. Organic milk is easy to find at supermarkets, because it has become such a popular product in the past five or so years. Research the livestock practices for the brand you choose; recently some large producers have been exposed in the press for running what amounts to dairy farm feedlots with thousands of cows living in poor conditions.

Butter and Cheese

When it comes to other dairy products, like cheese and butter, organic seems to be a better choice for another reason. Residues from many pesticides and herbicides are stored in fatty tissues and deposits in the bodies of cows (and other animals, including humans). Since most dairy products, such as butter, cream, and cheese, contain significant portions of fat, it's likely that consumption of nonorganic dairy products is an easy way for chemical and pesticide residues to get into your body.

In fact, one team of scientists has figured out that it's easier to track the levels of persistent organic pollutants (POP) simply by testing pats of butter from farms around the world than it is to use sophisticated monitoring equipment.[19] Toxic chemicals become concentrated in the fat in cow's milk, which is itself concentrated in butter. When you eat butter, environmental POPs become concentrated in your fat cells.

Recommendation: Organic butter and cheese may still be a little difficult to find in some areas, but they are worth seeking out so that you can avoid potential toxins concentrated in the fat. For foods that are eaten daily by children, like cottage cheese, cheese sticks, or cheese slices, it's wise to choose organic.

Eggs

Any moderately enlightened grocery store will carry white or brown eggs, "free-range" eggs, and "cage-free" eggs. Many stores also stock "organic" eggs, "fertile" eggs, and "fortified with omega-3" eggs. For the most discerning egg connoisseur, there are "pastured" eggs, which are typically only available directly from a farmer who raises chickens on grassy pastureland.

You should be aware that the organic label for eggs, as defined by the NOP standards, verifies only that neither the hens nor their feed were exposed to antibiotics, hormones, pesticides, or herbicides. None of the other claims made on egg packages—including "cage-free," "fertile," "all natural," or "farm fresh"—are regulated.

Given that, there are as many ways to raise hens as there are to cook an egg. Here's how to know which type of fresh egg is the best choice for your needs.

Conventional eggs are laid by hens in small cages that are stacked ceiling-high in a large temperature-controlled warehouse. Flocks of one 100,000 chickens are not uncommon. Pesticides can be used around the egg-production facility, in the feed, and even on the birds. The feed usually contains genetically modified corn and protein from animal by-products. The overwhelming majority of eggs laid in North America are from a single breed, the White Leghorn. There is very little genetic diversity in the world of commercial egg layers, and the risk of a devastating disease epidemic is significant. The chickens are thus given antibiotics to prevent diseases.

EGGS TO FIT YOUR PHILOSOPHY

"Organic" eggs come from chickens that are not given antibiotics or pesticides. The hens are fed corn, soybeans, and peas that were produced without pesticides, fungicides, herbicides, and are not from genetically modified seed stock. They typically have little access to the outdoors, because without antibiotics they are at greater risk for diseases. If you are pregnant, feeding a child, or want to avoid eggs from chickens exposed to pesticides, organic eggs are right for you.

"Cage-free organic" eggs are laid by hens that have some

access to the outdoors, but because they are not allowed to have antibiotics, outdoor roaming is really not encouraged. If you want organic eggs and you want the chicken who laid your eggs to know (but not necessarily experience) that there is a world outside their shed, these may the be eggs for you.

"Free-range" eggs come from hens that are fed conventional feed but are housed in sheds instead of cages and given room to roam in adjoining yards. Because of weather conditions, free-range hens are not actually raised outdoors, although they may be raised under less-crowded conditions. If you don't mind that the chickens that laid your eggs traded off eating genetically modified corn and antibiotics so that they could roam outside, peck bugs, and nest in boxes, free-range eggs will suit your philosophy.

EGGS FOR ROMANTIC VEGETARIANS WHO FAVOR DIVERSITY

"Fertile" eggs are from hens that live with a rooster. The myth that blood spots in eggs are from fertilization is not true. This harmless defect is from a tear in the hen's oviduct during egg formation and the eggs are perfectly safe to eat. If you're a true romantic, even where chickens are concerned, fertile eggs are right for you.

"Omega-3" eggs were developed to satisfy people's desire for diets that are higher in fish oil. Chicken feed is supplemented by fish oil and algae, so the eggs provide some fatty acids normally found in oily fish. These eggs can be organic or nonorganic. If you are a vegetarian and don't eat fish but want to increase your **HDL cholesterol**, omega-3 eggs are for you. These eggs are also popular with nonvegetarians who want more omega-3 fatty acids in their diet for the numerous health benefits.

Shell color is determined by the breed of chicken. Brown eggs mostly come from Rhode Island Red hens, which are often favored by organic farmers. White eggs come from White Leghorn chickens. Green, blue, and pink eggs come from Araucana and Ameraucana chickens, sometimes referred to as Easter Egg chickens. If you believe in diversity, selecting brown or green eggs casts a vote for genetic diversity among chickens.

THE CONNOISSEUR'S EGGS

Pastured hens are raised on grassy fields instead of being kept in confinement and fed grain-based chicken feed. Pastured hens eat grubs, bugs, earthworms, and other insects, which give their eggs a huge flavor boost. Pasturing is the old-fashioned way of raising hens and other poultry. It is a sustainable, humane method of raising chickens, and it produces the most delicious and nutritious eggs. Pastured eggs contain up to twenty times more omega-3 than other types of eggs; the bright orange yolks and the freshness create an egg with an incredible flavor.

Pastured egg farmers maintain open-air chicken roosts on wheels that they rotate through fields after the cows leave for greener pastures. The happy chickens peck the grubs and insects out of the pasture, thus minimizing the number of flies and insect pests on the farm. Pastured eggs are not necessarily organic just because they are part of a wild system, but the laying hens tend to be healthier than chickens raised in large production facilities. If you want the best-tasting eggs you've ever eaten, from chickens that wandered freely outdoors and pecked and ate freely, and you can get to a farm or farmers' market, pastured eggs are perfect.

Recommendation: Pastured eggs are well worth seeking out if you can find them (check www.localharvest.org or www.eatwellguide.org for a farm in your area). Otherwise, choose organic eggs to avoid potential residues from arsenic feed, antibiotics, and pesticides.

Chickens that lay cage-free organic eggs and organic eggs lead nearly identical lives, so if there is any difference between them, it is minimal. Organic omega-3 eggs are good choices for people who are trying to change their cholesterol profile and eat eggs regularly.

SEAFOOD

Currently the National Organic Standards Board has not developed or recommended meaningful organic standards for most fish and seafood. Almost all seafood, by its nature, comes from a wild and uncontrollable system, and the NOSB recognizes that an organic label would be impossible to verify. Although the organic certification of "wild-captured aquatic animals" would imply that entire ecosystems can be organic, the NOSB task force realized that "many critical management issues exceed the individual producer's influence" and in 2001 declined to create organic standards for fish.[20]

Although **aquaculture** could conceivably be managed as an organic system, farmed fish has already been shown to have many of the same environmental and health issues found on other large farm operations. Feed additives, antibiotics, and large areas of polluted water are the legacy of many aquaculture operations.

Strict fishing habitat management and sustainable fishing quotas are a better goal for fish producers than trying to shape organic standards to suit a wild product. The interests of consumers are best served if fish and seafood continue to come from wild sources that are managed well. At this point, "certified organic" seafood is simply a marketing tool for fish producers to capitalize on the trend to choose organic foods.

Recommendation: Buy wild seafood. Avoid farm-raised fish and prawns, and avoid fish labeled organic, as it is likely farm-raised fish. Be sure that your fish come from wild sources that are managed well to make certain that fish stocks are not depleted. If you are not certain what kind of fish your local market carries, ask them. They should be able to tell you if the fish is wild or farm-raised.

Nuts, Seeds, and Spices

Information about pesticide residues on nuts, seeds, and spices is not widely available, and sampling is not widely done on these foods. Most domestic tree nuts, such as walnuts and pecans, are sprayed with several preventive applications of pesticides, miticides, and herbicides. Tropical nuts, such as macadamias and cashews, are typically grown on smallish farms in countries like Vietnam, Brazil, and East Africa that don't use many pesticides. Unfortunately, the only pesticide residue information we have is from the EPA, and they lump all tree nuts together into a single category, which shows little pesticide residue.

A notable exception is almonds. The almond fruit looks similar to a small green peach (the nut grows inside like a peach pit), and the fruit, nut, and tree are attractive to many pests, nematodes, and diseases. Many highly toxic organophosphate pesticides and herbicides are approved for use in almond groves. Although organic almonds and almond butter can be expensive and difficult to find, organic almonds are worth seeking out, for both health reasons and environmental reasons.

The vast majority of sesame seeds, poppy seeds, and other seeds and spices are grown in developing countries where pesticides are not widely used for preventive measures.

Peanuts, which are actually legumes that grow underground, pick up toxic chemicals from the ground, including substances like DDT that have been banned for years. Alachlor, chlorothalonil, and methomyl are commonly used on peanut crops and are so toxic that in 2003 the attorneys general of New York, New Jersey, Massachusetts, and Connecticut sued the EPA for failing to protect children from the residues of these toxic pesticides on peanuts, peanut butter, and other foods.

Recommendation: Organic peanuts and peanut butter are highly recommended, especially for children who eat peanut butter frequently. If you eat almonds frequently, or if you are eating them for health reasons (for example, to increase HDL levels) you should find a source for organic almonds; the Internet may be the best place to look. One Internet source for almonds is Purity Organics (www.purity-organics.com) in California. If organic seeds are available and you eat them frequently (in bread, pastries, or tahini paste), it may be worth it to select organic. For occasional use, nonorganic seeds and spices are fine choices.

EDIBLE OILS

Most edible oils are processed extensively and heavily refined, so there is very little left of the original source of the oil. Organic oils may have more nutritional value (if they are unrefined), but there is not much, if any, pesticide residue in oil products. Buying organic oils does protect you against the effects of the GMO seed stock used for many oil-producing crops, such as canola (rapeseed), corn, and soybeans. GMO products are not identified as such in the United States, although other countries require that products containing GMO be labeled.

Olive groves, especially those in other countries, are not often sprayed with pesticides, primarily because that is not the custom, but also because their natural bitterness on the tree keeps potential pests away. Domestic olive oil from California is sprayed occasionally for olive flies, but trapping is also used to reduce reliance on pesticides.

Recommendation: It's a toss-up. Organic peanut and canola oils are better for the environment, but the health benefits are negligible. If you buy imported olive oil, it's unlikely to have been sprayed with pesticides. Organic olive oils are easy to find at most organic grocers and food co-ops.

Do avoid all partially hydrogenated fats such as shortening or margarine, even from organic sources, as these fats are unhealthy in any form.

GRAINS

Typically, grains are stripped of their outer husk, germ, and most of their nutrients to be processed into flour, rolled oats, and processed foods. After so much processing, little of the original surface area of the grain remains, and typically few pesticide residues are found in processed grains. A 2005 sampling of pesticide residues in the United Kingdom found that pesticide residues were more likely to be found in whole grain bread and cereals than in non-whole-grain products.

Rice grown in the United States always tests very high for pesticide residues, persistent organic pollutants, and some heavy metals. American-grown rice contains between 1.4 to 5 times more arsenic on average than rice from Europe, India, and Asia. Scientists think the likely reason stems from the American habit of growing rice on defunct cotton fields contaminated with long-banned arsenic pesticides.[21]

Recommendation: Buy organic rice whenever possible, or buy imported rice. For other grains, buy organic if you eat the entire grain, feed it to children, or eat it every day—oatmeal is a food that comes to mind.

Organic flour probably has no significant health benefit over nonorganic flour, but if there is little difference in price, organic is better for the environment and does not support the farm subsidy system. (For more information about the farm subsidy system, see page 71.)

SNACKS AND PROCESSED FOODS

Processed products such as bread, cereals, breakfast bars, chips, and cookies can be called organic if a majority of the ingredients are organic, but they do not have to be 100 percent organic to earn certification.

Most processed foods and snack foods have so many additives, preservatives, and flavorings, along with the highly processed flour, sugar, and high-fructose corn syrup in them, that buying them organic is not going to make you healthier. Even most so-called nutrition bars are highly processed amalgamations of dozens of ingredients, with little whole-food substance to them.

In most cases there is little, if any, health value in choosing organic processed foods, except perhaps to the environment. As discussed in chapter 1, many companies that make organic processed and snack foods are actually owned by large companies like General Mills, Kellogg, Kraft, and M&M/Mars (see page 10).

Although there are notable exceptions, such as Newman's Own Organics and Annie's Homegrown Mac & Cheese, often the organic grocery dollars you spend on snacks and processed foods are going right back to big-business producers.

Recommendation: Read the ingredients list to see exactly what ingredients are organic, and buy processed food organics only when cost is no object. However, if the food is something that children eat a lot of, whether it's boxed instant noodles, breakfast bars, dry cereals, or cookies, it's wise to buy organic.

SUMMING UP:
SOME FINAL SUGGESTIONS

1. If it's something you or your children eat or drink every day, like milk, butter, or cereal, try to buy organic.
2. If a child can eat a large portion in one sitting, for instance, of strawberries, buy organic.
3. If it's one of the Dirty Dozen (see chapter 6) fruits or vegetables, always buy organic.
4. Most tropical fruits are low in pesticide residue, so conventionally grown products are generally okay.
5. Fruits with thick rinds or peels are often low in pesticide residues, as long as you don't eat the peel, so choosing nonorganic versions is fine.
6. If you eat meat, try to find a source for sustainably raised meat products or organic meats.
7. It's not worth paying a premium for organic fish or seafood, but local wild fish and seafood will always be better than farm-raised.
8. Buying locally from a farmer you can talk with about production methods is a good alternative to buying organics.

·8·

where to find healthy food

MOST CONSUMERS who purchase organics are highly aware that in-season, locally grown, organic, sustainable Fair Trade food is the best choice. Sounds good, right? Now just try to find it, for everything you want to buy, all year round.

More often, shoppers are confronted with several less than desirable choices—produce that has traveled thousands of miles to get to the store, organic produce that duplicates the big-business way of production, or conventionally grown local food. If you have concerns about the distance traveled, the production method, and the seasonality of your food, you may have to work around the typical ways that food is distributed and sold.

More and more farmers and shoppers are finding ways to circumvent the traditional economic route for food distribution. Some small farmers have built such strong relationships with customers that they no longer sell to distributors, grocery stores, or even farmers' markets. Dedicated customers come directly to the farm, or they buy invitation-only CSA shares in a farm. These farmers send customers weekly e-mails or electronic newsletters to keep them informed about the farm's progress, what foods are available, and how to make a purchase.

These economic paths allow customers to ask farmers direct questions, such as "Why are your vegetables more expensive than the vegetables in the supermarket? Shouldn't organic foods be cheaper, since you don't have to pay for expensive chemicals?" And it allows the farmer to answer, "Because of their dangers, I use no pesticides or chemical fertilizers on my farm, so my yields are lower; no workers on my farm are paid less than minimum wage; and my vegetables taste better than anything you can buy at the supermarket."[1]

Yes, you do pay a premium to buy food that is grown or raised in a sustainable, ethical manner. However, for a growing number of people who care about not only where their food comes from but also the ecological footprint it leaves on the earth, that premium seems worth paying.

The following sections are included to provide you with ideas about where you can find healthy foods, both organic and nonorganic. These options are presented as general guidelines, based on my experiences, and are not ranked.

WHOLE FOODS AND WILD OATS:
ORGANIC SHOPPING MADE EASY

If you want to select from the entire spectrum of organic and natural food offerings, you just can't beat Whole Foods and Wild Oats Markets. Not only do they have a selection that is unsurpassed by other stores, but they also have high ethical standards for selecting food (particularly seafood and meat) and are political advocates for organic standards. These stores and other natural grocery stores cater to the "organic lifestyle" shopper.

* Whole Foods, with sales of $4.7 billon in 2005, is by far the largest natural foods grocer, with 187 stores in the United States and the United Kingdom.
* Wild Oats, a national chain headquartered in Boulder, Colorado, is second, reporting sales of $1.1 billion from 110 stores in 2005.
* At Wild Oats, 70 percent of the produce and 40 percent of the packaged food is organic.

Although Whole Foods does not publish exact ratios (and that ratio naturally changes from summer to winter), they seem to stock slightly more organic than conventional food. At both stores you'll find a wide selection of high-quality fresh foods, along with organic staples like pasta, cereal, and cooking oils, as well as full-service meat, cheese, seafood, bakery, and floral departments. You'll also find a full spectrum of herbal and nutritional supplements, and environmentally friendly household cleaners and paper products. Both stores have a gourmet deli filled with ready-to-eat organic meals that range from organic rotisserie chickens to vegetarian salads, seasoned tofu, and vegan or raw food entrées.

Whole Foods and Wild Oats are stores where you can spend your afternoon browsing, sampling foods, and filling up your cart. Before you know it, you may find yourself forking over three hundred dollars for a cart of organic groceries. Ouch! That's why Whole Foods has earned the unwelcome, but apt, nickname "Whole Paycheck." With posters of happy, apple-cheeked farmers standing in their fields of green over the produce section, along with soft lighting and helpful employees, they make shoppers feel virtuous while they spend money.

Recent articles in *The New Yorker* and other media have criticized Whole Foods for giving shoppers the illusion that shopping there supports small farmers. The reality is that a small farmer would not be able to keep up with the demand of even one Whole Foods store. Whole Foods stocks much more conventional produce than their advertising and in-store marketing would suggest, and they also buy produce from huge organic farms in the United States, China, and other countries.

If you can buy directly from small farmers, you should. When you cannot, Whole Foods and Wild Oats are good places to shop, browse, and explore organic and natural foods.

Advantages: Convenient hours and locations; wide selection; high-quality organic and conventional produce; ready-to-eat organic deli foods; feels similar to a conventional grocery store experience.

Disadvantages: It's easy to overspend; most items have traveled a long distance to the store.

FOOD CO-OPS AND NATURAL FOOD STORES: CONTRIBUTING TO THE LOCAL ECOMONY

Food cooperatives and natural food stores are independent groceries where most, if not all, of the fruits and vegetables are organic. Many co-ops buy from local farmers on a regular basis, although most also purchase produce from distributors. Co-ops often have a membership fee, or they may require members to work at the co-op for a few hours each month. There are about 150 food co-ops presently operating in the United States[2] (see Resources) and over a dozen operating in Canada.

I'll never forget bringing my mother, who was visiting from Michigan, along with me to our local food cooperative in

Seattle. As I shopped, she was looking around at the produce, bulk food bins, rows of vitamins, and wide selection of goat cheeses. I thought she was finding the experience an interesting contrast to the bland, plastic-filled grocery stores back home. But when it was time to check out, she told me she had actually been looking around for a six-pack of Coke but couldn't find any. "Mom," I said, "they don't sell Coke here."

"No Coke?" she said, her eyes widening as she shook her head in disbelief.

Advantages: Connection to local economy; convenient locations; fresher organic produce (co-ops), meats, chicken, and dairy than conventional groceries; they often sell local baked goods; ready-to-eat organic deli food.

Disadvantages: More expensive than conventional grocery stores; sorry, Mom—no Cokes or other common grocery store brand-name items like chewing gum, cereals, salad dressings, and toothpaste, although they often have organic versions of such products.

FARMERS' MARKETS, U-PICK, FARM STANDS:
THE FRESH CHOICE

The farmers' market movement in the United States has been growing dramatically since the 1980s, with the number of farmers' markets more than doubling from 1994 to 2004.[3] Now there are more than four thousand farmers' markets across the country. Shopping at the farmers' market brings you closer to nature, closer to your community, and closer to your food. People take the time to chat with the farmers, cheese makers, beekeepers, and bakers, and they can ask a lot of questions.

Every Sunday morning my daughter and I head over to what looks like a street fair. Music is playing, colorful banners are flying in the breeze, tables are piled high with food and flowers, and people are milling around. It's our neighborhood farmers' market, and though it fills only about one-half of a city block, the market is a summertime destination. I love to look around and see shoppers and farmers, teenagers and parents, grandparents and little kids, talking about food, eating food, carrying flats of fruits and bunches of vegetables. Seeing shoppers and vendors talking and laughing together, it seems clear that farmers' markets really put the "culture" back in agriculture.

When you buy food directly from a farmer, most of the money goes back to the farm instead of to distributors, shippers, and grocery stores. You can find the established farmers' markets in your area by looking on the Internet (www.localharvest.org or www.eatwellguide.org).

Advantages: Fresh, mostly organic seasonal food; low prices; connection with farms and local community; opportunity to ask questions.

Disadvantages: You probably cannot purchase everything you need for a meal; many farmers' markets operate only once or twice a week for a few hours, and the short hours may not work for your schedule. The Greenmarket at Union Square in New York City (which operates Monday, Wednesday, Friday, and Saturday), the Ferry Terminal Market in San Francisco, the Pike Place Market in Seattle, and a handful of other markets are open every day or nearly every day.

The Crescent City Farmers' Market of New Orleans

This is the story of how Poppy Tooker (and her many allies) saved Thanksgiving 2004 for New Orleans by reviving the Crescent City Farmers' Market. If you were anywhere in America on August 29, 2004, you remember the terrible images of New Orleans swamped by seawater after Hurricane Katrina hit. Thousands of city residents trapped in the city were left to fend for themselves by inept government agencies, and more than 1,800 people died as a result of the storm and the subsequent flooding.

Poppy doesn't even like to say the K word, and I imagine that if you lived through the total devastation of your beloved city, you wouldn't want to give it a cute nickname, either. "I am determined that the rest of my life is not going to be about this," she says with a long sigh, "and I just, I just don't even want the word used." She simply refers to it as "the storm."

Poppy, a cooking teacher, had started a Slow Food convivium in New Orleans in 1999. (Slow Food began in 1989 as a movement to preserve the regional cuisine and associated crops, livestock, and preservation methods of those regions. See www.slowfood.com for more information about the Slow Food movement.) The convivium ended up providing critical support to New Orleans farmers after the hurricane hit. "When I formed the convivium here, we were immediately captivated by the idea of the Arc of Taste [a Slow Food phrase that refers to traditional foods and methods of preservation that are threatened by mass production.]. One of my partners in that endeavor was the Crescent City Farmers' Market. We began to nominate foods that we regarded as endangered in our culture—things like Creole cream cheese and the Louisiana tangi berry [similar to a strawberry]—for inclusion. We worked hand-in-hand with the farmers.

"Then, along comes the storm. In the very first days after the storm, Richard McCarthy [the market's founder] and I were able to get in touch, although he was in Houston. I remember hearing Richard's sad voice saying, 'Poppy, our whole food distribution system is going to be broken. It's so broken and I don't know what we're going to do.'"

Poppy, who returned to New Orleans shortly after the storm hit, immediately went to work to fix that broken system. "In the early days after the storm, the first few brave souls who were trying to reopen their restaurants didn't have any access to food," she says. "So we set up a crazy distribution system where I was contacting farmers and then telling restaurant chefs what the farmers had to sell." The farmers would designate a driver to make a weekly delivery to Poppy's cooking school, The Savvy Gourmet, on Magazine Street. The chefs would pick up food and leave money for the farmers in an envelope. "I was really bewildered," she said. "My sister-in-law had one empty bedroom, so me, my husband, my daughter, and our dog were living in one bedroom. You can't imagine how difficult it was to focus on what needed to be done."

Meanwhile, New Orleans was still in total shambles, as were the lives of many of its residents. Because seawater had seeped into the ground for so long, all of the vegetation had died. "The city looked like it had been nuked," she recollects. "All the magnolia trees were dead. The grass was brown. The landscape was horrifically stark. We were all alone. For weeks and weeks, we were the only people living on our block."

In the weeks after the storm, no grocery stores were open, so Poppy had to make a two-hour round trip to Baton Rouge for food. Finally, in mid-October, after six weeks two grocery stores finally reopened, with nearly bare shelves and no fresh food.

"I'll never forget this," says Poppy. "When the stores opened, I would go to both stores every single day to try to buy butter, which is my comfort food. But all they had were squeeze bottles of margarine," she remembers. "After days and days of trying to buy a single stick of butter, I finally just broke down. I was standing there in the dairy section, crying. I was crying to see what had become of my city."

In spite of her own struggles, when Poppy heard that market vendors Ray and Kay Brandhurst and their four children had lost their shrimp boat, their home, and their business in the storm, she tried to help them. "They had lost everything," she said. "Their families had lost everything. His shrimp boat had sunk."

Poppy e-mailed the Brandhursts to see how she could help them recover from the storm. Kay's eloquent e-mail reply, which spoke to her desire to save her family's culture and livelihood despite the storm, touched Poppy deeply. She forwarded the e-mail to her Slow Food friends, who quickly raised money to help Brandhurst and other farmers recover from the destruction caused by Katrina.

Meanwhile, Poppy, Richard, and others continued working to reopen the farmers' market for residents who were coming back to a devastated city. Amazingly, the market reopened on the Tuesday before Thanksgiving, only ten weeks after the storm hit. The Brandhursts' boat had been raised, the motors were running, and Kay was at the market with a big load of shrimp to sell. Several farmers came with whatever they had to sell, along with a fisherman and a couple of bakers with homemade Thanksgiving pies and cookies—all of whom were greeted by plenty of excited customers.

The food from the farmers' market allowed the Tooker family, the Brandhurst family, and many other families in New Orleans to enjoy a Thanksgiving dinner that year. "There was nothing good at the grocery stores. It was terrible," says Poppy. "To have Thanksgiving dinner, to enjoy our traditional foods— the farmers' market was the only way."

"It felt like a miracle," she remembers. "That was the happiest, happiest day in New Orleans since August twenty-ninth—when the farmers' market opened [for business again]. It was a beautiful sunny, cold day, and it felt like a great homecoming. Here in New Orleans—and I'm sure this is true in other parts of the country—the farmers' market really feeds our spirit and our soul. The farmers' market is our community."

CRESCENT CITY FARMERS' MARKET
When: Tuesdays/year-round/rain or shine, 9 A.M. to 1 P.M.
Where: 200 Broadway (the Uptown Square parking lot)
New Orleans, Louisiana
For more information: www.crescentcityfarmersmarket.org

COMMUNITY-SUPPORTED AGRICULTURE (CSA):
A FRESH INVESTMENT IN FARMS

Another way to buy direct from the farmer is to buy shares in a CSA program. A CSA is like a subscription, or an investment, in a farm. People offer their consistent support to the farm's operation so that the farmland becomes, either legally or in spirit, a farm that belongs to its members. The farmer and the customers share ideas and support, as well as sharing the risks and benefits of farming.

Typically, you pay one lump sum (or several installment payments) to a farmer in the spring to cover the anticipated costs of the farm operation and farmer's salary. Through direct sales, farmers receive better prices for their crops, gain financial flexibility, and do not have to be as concerned with marketing their produce.

In return, customers receive a basket of mixed fresh produce every week throughout the growing season. Most CSA shares are offered in small and large sizes for different-size families; you might share one with a neighbor or friend if you cannot use up that much produce in one week.

CSA shares offer the opportunity to have a direct relationship with a local farmer; support a local organic or sustainable farm; and share the harvest of fruits, vegetables, and herbs (sometimes flowers) each week. CSA members also share in the risks of farming, including poor harvests due to drought, floods or insect problems. If your farm experiences a poor growing season, your CSA share will be small.

Advantages: Very fresh, mostly organic seasonal food; low cost; the opportunity to build a relationship with a farm; you often receive heirloom varietals (uncommon plant varieties that have survived for generations because of the preservation efforts of individuals) and other rare gems not sold at stores; larger harvests can mean bonus produce for shareholders.

Disadvantages: You get what they are picking that week, with no substitutions; you have to pick up the boxes at a certain day, time, and location; produce not picked up (due to vacation, emergency, etc.) is usually donated to a local food bank—no refunds.

THE HOME-DELIVERY BOX:
ORGANICS AT YOUR DOORSTEP

Organic home-delivery services (such as Diamond Organics, Fresh Direct, Small Potatoes, and Planet Organics) have filled in part of the niche left hanging when many of the online grocery-delivery services went bankrupt in the late 1990s. They offer a box of organic produce, much like a CSA, but they deliver it to your door once a week or ship it overnight.

Home-delivery services have a Web site where you can make changes to the contents of your box or order additional groceries. Most services do not allow you to completely customize your box, but they typically allow two or three substitutions. Many home-delivery services have widened their selection to include organic pastas and snacks, baby food, and even dairy and meat products. If you have few options for organic produce, or if you are too busy to shop, home-delivery services can meet your needs.

Be aware that home-delivery services sometimes trim costs by buying discounted "Grade B" produce that cannot be sold in grocery stores because it's too ripe (like melons or berries) or too small (like mushrooms or apples). However, most are happy to credit you for items that are not up to your standards.

Advantages: They deliver to your door; reasonable cost; they allow limited customization of your box; many support local farmers and producers.

Disadvantages: If you are not home for the delivery, the box may sit in front of your door for several hours; some produce may not be up to standards; typically it's difficult to change delivery day and time.

CONVENTIONAL GROCERY STORES: CONVENIENCE THAT'S HARD TO BEAT

Most grocery stores carry some organic food, even if it's only packaged foods like Ragu Organic Spaghetti Sauce or Annie's Homegrown Organic Noodles and Cheese. Some of them even have well-stocked organic produce and dairy sections. In other grocery stores the selection is limited to foods with long storage potential, such as ultra-pasteurized milk, apples, oranges, and bagged lettuces. Groceries are very sensitive to customer demand, so the more organic shoppers in your area, the more likely you are to find a wide variety of organic products.

Prices for organic foods in season are sometimes comparable to prices of the same items that have been conventionally grown—particularly herbs, salad greens, bananas, scallions, and apples. It's worth browsing the organic produce section to see if you can pick up organics, especially for foods like apples and strawberries that are favorites of children. Newman's Own Organics products, which include fresh juices and cookies (foods that some children consume in large quantities), are also found in many mainstream groceries.

Advantages: Always open; in your neighborhood; generally a good selection of products; prices are reasonable.

Disadvantages: Selection of organic foods is limited, but they often have the basics; little or no purchasing from local farmers.

Costco and Wal-Mart:
A SURPRISING NEW SOURCE FOR ORGANICS

When I started working on this book, I never thought that these huge discount stores would be options for buying organic produce. But as of 2006, both have moved assertively into the organics market and now sell hundreds of organic products. "Sustainable" and "free trade" have crept into Wal-Mart corporate lingo alongside "everyday low prices." You know that when Costco and Wal-Mart start selling something, it has really made its way into the consciousness of Middle America.

The quality of the organic produce in these stores is good, and the prices tend to be lower than most other retail outlets for organic foods. Sometimes the reason for the low prices is that produce is imported from China and other countries (see pages 53). As a result, the organic produce may suffer in quality compared to other sources. You may also have to purchase larger quantities than you really want in order to see the discount (such as an entire flat of berries or bag of apples). Milk products are generally ultrapasteurized for long shelf life. Overall you can find many organic products at a discount if a low price is your main priority

Advantages: Low prices; convenient hours and locations.

Disadvantages: Discount stores often sell only large quantities (like ten-pound bags of organic apples) that are not always desirable for perishables; selection varies; little or no purchasing from local farmers.

Ten Tips for Eating Healthy Food
Even if You're Not Wealthy

∾

1. Shop the farmers' markets for food in season. The best prices and the freshest organic produce come from the farmers' market.

2. Buy seasonal produce in large quantities and freeze what you cannot use immediately. You can make shakes and smoothies all winter from a couple flats of frozen organic strawberries or raspberries. The flavor is better, too!

3. Shop around at different stores to see where the values are found. Plan your shopping trips around your findings.

4. Join a food co-op. Members often receive a discount or monthly coupon for 5–10 percent discounts.

5. Buy a share in a CSA. Shares are typically about four hundred dollars (you can pay installments) for a weekly box of produce during the growing season. The cost typically works out to about thirty dollars or less per week.

6. Use coupons. The best way to obtain coupons for natural or organic foods is to visit the Web site of the manufacturer, or use an Internet search engine and type in the words "grocery store coupons" and "organic" for printable coupons.

7. Buy from the bulk bins. Organic flour, sugar, cereals, pasta, spices, and many snack foods are less

expensive (and easier on the environment) if you purchase them from the bulk food section. Some stores even have peanut butter, maple syrup, cooking oil, and even cleaning products available in bulk. Bring your reusable bags or containers and reduce your waste at the same time.

8. Grow your own healthy foods.

9. Shop the sales. Buy organic or shade-grown coffee beans on sale and freeze the excess. Organic meats, frozen foods, butter, and bread products all freeze well for several months.

10. Practice cooking creatively. When you have leftovers from dinner, try to use them in another meal—add them to a pasta dish, veggie burrito, or omelet, or fold them into a soup or sauce. Don't waste food.

GROWING YOUR OWN FOOD:
THE ENJOYMENT OF GOING BACK TO NATURE ON YOUR OWN

Food from your own garden is a very inexpensive way to eat pesticide-free foods. Many fruits and vegetables, even fruit trees, can be grown successfully in containers or in small, urban spaces.

Growing your own food is as local as you can possibly get, and at the same time it's an enjoyable and fulfilling activity. I mix a few bean plants, cucumber vines, and tomato plants into my perennial beds in early spring and harvest a few handfuls of each by late summer. The plants add seasonal interest to my garden beds, and the vegetables are a nice bonus. Children especially get much pleasure from planting seeds and watching them grow. It seems important that city children realize that food grows in the earth, in the dirt, and that it doesn't just come from a grocery store. Be sure to avoid fertilizing with nonorganic chicken manure or steer manure, because it is likely to contain contaminants.

Another bonus is that sometimes when kids are involved in growing vegetables they are more likely to eat them. I wondered when my young daughter would ever eat a green vegetable until the year that I grew shelling peas. One day she and her little friends started pulling them off the vines and eating the peas. I vowed to grow peas every year from then on, and she still loves them.

Now that she's five years old, I let her choose vegetables when we go to the farmers' market. Her tastes run a little exotic—she favors peppercress, radicchio, and the occasional conjoined-twin squash, cucumber, or pumpkin. I keep hoping that one day she'll take a big bite of that peppercress, begin to eat lots of vegetables, and never turn back. And I think it's going to happen.

Community gardens (see Resources) are another way to grow your own foods. Many cities have fenced spaces set aside where residents can plant almost anything they can grow. Sometimes the spaces are free, and sometimes there is a nominal fee for water and compost.

Advantages: High level of control over production methods; low cost; greater connection to your food; if you enjoy gardening, it can be a very pleasant hobby.

Disadvantages: Production is limited by the size of your garden space; it make take a few seasons to figure out what grows best in your garden; dirt under your fingernails (gardening gloves can help here).

• afterword •

Organic and sustainable food always seems to look better and taste better to me. I don't know if that's because it's usually fresher or if it's the way the food is grown, but I can always taste the difference between organic lettuce and conventionally grown lettuce.

I go to the farmers' market every Sunday (even in the winter), with my five-year-old daughter in tow. We make a game of counting how many vegetables she can name correctly, or playing I Spy as we walk around the lively market. I want to make sure she grows up with an enthusiasm for good food and that she understands the hard work it takes to grow that food.

Making an effort to connect to your local food network has a long-term value. I always make a point to converse with the farmers and their families who work at the farmers' market. They have educated me, and thousands of other market-goers, about organic growing and sustainable farming. Why do the cucumbers they grow taste so amazing? Why are there so few eggs available in the summer? How do they make their peaches taste like juicy, sweet, dripping slices of sunlight?

Over and over again they tell me the same thing: "This was grown in the right soil, under the right conditions, and picked this morning. You really don't need to do anything to make it taste great. Mother Nature has already done the work."

THE ARTISAN FARMER:
PRODUCING FOOD AND BUILDING
RELATIONSHIPS THE OLD-FASHIONED WAY

Well, farmers can be a little *too* modest. Farming is hard work. In the process of writing this book, I've talked with many farmers, including organic growers, sustainable farmers, and nonorganic farmers. Despite the toil of farming, they all find their work deeply satisfying and fulfilling. Just as a chef is happy knowing that someone out in the dining room is swooning over the meal she prepared, a farmer is happy knowing that he selected the right plant; gave it rich soil, water, and sunshine; and harvested it at the perfect moment to make it to your table.

Many farmers want to talk with customers about their crops, about the chickens they raise or the cows they milk. They can tell you how to cook the food they grow, when certain foods will be in season, or why their cows' milk tastes sweeter in the spring. All you need to do is let them know you are interested and start the conversation. Close the gap between you and the people who grow your food by asking them questions, talking about the weather (farmers are obsessed with the weather), and letting them know what you think about their offerings.

As I spoke with Poppy Tooker (see Crescent City Farmers Market, page 141), and Amy Hepworth (see Hepworth Farms, page 28), and others involved with producing food in this country, I learned a lot about small farms. I also came to understand that it is critically important for all of us as consumers to have contacts with local farms and to know the farmers who live nearby.

I've made that point throughout this book and given you many reasons to connect with farmers, but here's a big one: if you are ever unfortunate enough to live through a disaster like Hurricane Katrina, or a 9/11, an earthquake or tsunami, a mad cow or food bacteria scare—or that "pandemic" the politicians are always warning us about—clearly, you can not depend on the government to restore order and feed you immediately. We should all realize that by now. It's more likely to be the people in your town, in your neighborhood, and at your farmers' market, or greengrocer, who will be able to supply what you and your family need to survive. Even if you're a very busy person, slow it down once in a while and take a drive to a local farm, just so you know where it's located.

GOING ORGANIC:
START LIVING HEALTHIER TODAY

Greengrocers, natural food markets, and food cooperatives are the next closest step to buying direct from the farmer. Many people work in these markets because they have a passion for food. Talk with the produce stocker or your cashier about what looks good that week. Question them about where their produce is grown, or ask them how they like to cook kale and leeks. Don't be shy. It's your food, your body, and your family. You have to seek out and support the people in your community who care about growing, raising, and selling the best food that nature can provide.

Whether you decide to buy or not to buy organic food when you shop for groceries, one thing is for certain: produce that is trucked thousands of miles and stacked in a chilly supermarket aisle will never taste as fresh as produce that was picked a few hours ago or even a few days ago. Making the effort to connect with the farmers who grow your food—whether it's through farmers' markets, farm stands, community-supported agriculture shares, or U-pick farms—is the best way you can enrich your diet and improve your health.

• Shopping Guide •

FOOD	BUY ORGANIC	NOT ORGANIC	LOCAL	CHEW ON THIS . . .
Almonds	✳			Many toxic pesticides and herbicides are used on almond trees. If you are eating almonds daily for health reasons (for example, to improve your cholesterol), you should buy organic almonds.
Apples	✳			Multiple pesticides are found on apples, a favorite food of many children. Buy organic.
Apricots	✳			Like most stone fruits, apricots are highly likely to contain pesticide residues. Organic is recommended.

FOOD	BUY ORGANIC	NOT ORGANIC	LOCAL	CHEW ON THIS ...
Asparagus		✳		Asparagus does not appeal to many insect pests. Nonorganic asparagus rarely contains pesticide residue and is a fine choice.
Avocados		✳		Low pesticide residues and a thick skin make nonorganic avocados an acceptable choice.
Baby Food	✳			Make your own or buy only 100% organic baby food.
Baby Formula	✳			Organic formula is best. You may have to look for it on the Internet. Itspoils more quickly than does nonorganic formula, so don't overstock.
Bananas		✳		Low pesticide residues and a thick skin make nonorganic bananas an acceptable choice. Free trade bananas or organic bananas are often the same price as nonorganic.
Basil	✳			Leafy greens that grow close to the ground tend to have higher pesticide residues than other vegetables. Organic basil is often available year-round.

FOOD	BUY ORGANIC	NOT ORGANIC	LOCAL	CHEW ON THIS . . .
Beans, dried		✳	✳	Beans are typically sprayed with several insecticides to prevent insects and their larvae from damaging the crop. There is not much testing data on dried beans, and they are lumped together into one catergory by the PDP. Beans are typically washed, soaked, rinsed, and then boiled, so it is likely that residues are removed in the process.
Beef	✳			If you cannot buy organic, grass-fed beef, stick to leaner cuts, as pesticide residue is stored in fat.
Beets	✳			Thin-skinned vegetables that grow underground can absorb pesticides and heavy metals. Organic is best.
Bell Peppers, all colors		✳		Always buy organic peppers. Conventionally grown peppers are highly likely to contain pesticide residues.
Blackberries			✳	Blackberries have low pesticide residues. Quality will be best from a local grower.

FOOD	BUY ORGANIC	NOT ORGANIC	LOCAL	CHEW ON THIS . . .
Blueberries			✳	Blueberries have low pesticide residues. Quality will be best from a local grower.
Bread			✳	Bread is so processed that very little of the wheat grain is left. Organic is great if you can find it, especially for children. Quality will be best from a local bakery.
Broccoli		✳		Pesticides don't work well, so few are used.
Brussels Sprouts		✳		Pesticides don't work well, so few are used.
Butter	✳			Buy organic if price is no object. Butter shows low pesticide levels typically, but pesticide residues are stored in fat and butter is nearly all fat.
Cabbage		✳		Pesticides don't work well, so few are used.
Cantaloupe, from Mexico		✳		Imported cantaloupes have more pesticide residue. A better choice is domestic conventional or organic melons.

FOOD	BUY ORGANIC	NOT ORGANIC	LOCAL	CHEW ON THIS...
Carrots	✳			Carrots are so good at absorbing heavy metals from soil, they are sometimes grown as a throwaway crop to rid a field of lead or arsenic contamination. Buy only organic carrots, especially for children.
Cashews		✳		Cashews are grown almost exclusively in tropical locations where pesticides are rarely used.
Cauliflower		✳		Pesticides don't work well, so few are used.
Celery	✳			Celery readily absorbs everything from the soil, including plenty of pesticides. Nonorganic celery is the vegetable most likely to contain pesticide residues: 82% of samples were positive. Buy only organic.
Cheese	✳		✳	Cheese is mostly fat, and pesticides and persistent organic pollutants tend to accumulate in animal fat. Organic cheese is best, but admittedly hard to find. For cheese sticks that children eat regularly, buy only organic. Local cheese makers may be a good option.

FOOD	BUY ORGANIC	NOT ORGANIC	LOCAL	CHEW ON THIS . . .
Cherries	✳			Cherries are sprayed 8–10 times during the growth cycle with various pesticides and other chemicals. As a result, they are highly likely to contain pesticide residue. Buy only organic. Bottled or canned cherries have a lower pesticide load if organic is not available.
Chicken	✳			Especially for babies, small children, and people who eat chicken frequently, organic chicken is recommended because of the arsenic in nonorganic chicken meat.
Chicken Livers	✳			The liver metabolizes toxins, and chicken livers have 2–4 times the arsenic levels of muscle tissue. If you eat large amounts of chicken liver, choose organic livers.
Chocolate		✳		After processing, pesticide residues are not typically found in chocolate. Free trade chocolate is good for the farmers.

FOOD	BUY ORGANIC	NOT ORGANIC	LOCAL	CHEW ON THIS . . .
Cilantro		*		Cilantro grows quickly and is rarely sprayed with pesticides, although herbicides are sprayed early in the growth cycle to kill competing weeds. Nonorganic cilantro is acceptable.
Collard Greens	*			Leafy greens that grow close to the ground tend to have high pesticide residue levels. Buy organic.
Cookies	*			If your children eat something everyday, or almost every day, make it organic. Buy cookies that do not contain partially hydrogenated fat, as trans fat is unsafe for humans.
Cooking Oil		*		Not much of the original grain, fruit, or nut is left after oil extraction, so oils have little pesticide residue. Organic oils are not grown from GMO seed stock and are better for the environment. If price is no object, buy organic.

FOOD	BUY ORGANIC	NOT ORGANIC	LOCAL	CHEW ON THIS . . .
Corn, Sweet			✳	Although it is sprayed with herbicides and some pesticides, sweet corn almost never contains pesticide residue. Local corn always tastes best.
Cucumbers	✳			Highly toxic organophosphate pesticides are used on conventionally grown cukes. Only buy organic.
Daikon Radishes		✳		Daikon radishes do not appeal to most insects, and few pesticides or herbicides are used on this crop. Conventional is acceptable.
Eggplant, all varieties		✳		Although it is sprayed with pesticides and herbicides, eggplant rarely contains pesticide residue. Conventional eggplant is acceptable.
Eggs	✳		✳	Local pastured eggs are wonderful if you have access to a farm. If not, organic eggs are the next best choice, followed by cage-free eggs.

FOOD	BUY ORGANIC	NOT ORGANIC	LOCAL	CHEW ON THIS...
Figs	✳			Many highly toxic pesticides are used on figs. These thin-skinned fruits are not widely tested for pesticide residue, but are likely to contain residue. Organic figs are best when you can find them.
Garlic		✳		Garlic has natural pest control and is rarely sprayed with pesticides. Nonorganic garlic has few, if any, pesticide residues.
Ginger		✳		Like most tropical plants grown for food, ginger is rarely sprayed with pesticides or herbicides, if at all. Nonorganic ginger is acceptable.
Grapefruit		✳		Among citrus fruits, grapefruit rank the lowest in pesticide residue. The peel is where most pesticide residue is concentrated, so buy organic when using the peel.
Grapes, domestic		✳		Grapes grown in the U.S. typically test low for pesticide residue. Nonorganic grapes are fine, but for small children, organic is the best choice.

FOOD	BUY ORGANIC	NOT ORGANIC	LOCAL	CHEW ON THIS . . .
Grapes, imported	✳			Buy only organic or avoid imported grapes entirely, especially for children. Imported grapes are fumigated with methyl bromide, a highly toxic and dangerous ozone-depleting chemical.
Green Beans	✳			Green beans are sprayed multiple times with pesticides, herbicides, and fungicides. Buy only organic.
Green Onions		✳		Onions have natural pest control; green onions are sometimes sprayed with an herbicide early in the growth cycle. Organic is better, but nonorganic is acceptable.
Juice	✳			Juices test lower than fresh fruits for pesticide residue. For young children, organics are the best choice.
Kale	✳			Leafy greens that grow close to the ground tend to have high pesticide residue levels. Buy organic.

FOOD	BUY ORGANIC	NOT ORGANIC	LOCAL	CHEW ON THIS . . .
Ketchup	*			Organic tomato products contain more of the cancer-fighting carotenoid lycopene. Choose organic if available.
Leeks		*		Although they are typically sprayed with pesticides and herbicides, nonorganic leeks have few pesticide residues.
Lemons	*			The peel is where most pesticide residue is concentrated, so buy organic when using the peel for baking or drinks.
Lettuce	*			Leafy greens that grow close to the ground tend to have high pesticide residue levels. Buy organic.
Limes	*			The peel is where most pesticide residue is concentrated, so buy organic when using the peel for baking or drinks.
Macadamia Nuts		*		Few pesticides, if any are typically used on macadamia nuts.

FOOD	BUY ORGANIC	NOT ORGANIC	LOCAL	CHEW ON THIS . . .
Macaroni & Cheese, boxed	✳			Even though it's a processed food with low pesticide residues, if children eat it more than once a week, buy organic.
Mandarin Oranges		✳		Mandarin oranges typically have the lowest amount of pesticide residues of all citrus fruits.
Mangoes		✳		This thick-sklinned tropical fruit has little or no pesticide residue. Nonorganic mangos are acceptable.
Milk	✳			Organic milk does not contain hormones or antibiotics, which is why many people choose it. Some organic milk producers run dairy farms like factory farms, so research the brand of milk you buy carefully. Organic milk is highly recommended.
Mint	✳			The highly toxic organophosphate malaithon is used as a pesticide on commercial mint. Organic is the best choice.

FOOD	BUY ORGANIC	NOT ORGANIC	LOCAL	CHEW ON THIS . . .
Napa Cabbage	✳			Always buy organic. Napa cabbage is sprayed with several organophosphate pesticides, fungicides, and herbicides. It is highly likely to contain residues after harvest.
Nectarines	✳			Like most stone fruits, nectarines are highly likely to contain multiple pesticide residues. Organic is recommended, especially for children.
Oatmeal	✳			If you eat oatmeal every day, or if you eat it for health benefits, or if you feed it to children, organic oatmeal is recommended.
Okra		✳		Few pesticides are approved or needed to grow okra successfully. Hot, hot weather is the most important factor. Nonorganic okra is a fine choice.
Onions		✳		Onions and other members of the allium family have natural pest control and are not sprayed much. Nonorganic onions have few pesticide residues.

FOOD	BUY ORGANIC	NOT ORGANIC	LOCAL	CHEW ON THIS . . .
Oranges	✳			The peel is where most pesticide residue is concentrated, so buy organic when using the peel for baking or drinks.
Orange Juice		✳		Orange juice tests lower than fresh oranges for pesticide residues, but still contains some. Nonorganic is acceptable but, for children, organic is better.
Papayas		✳		Thick-skinned tropical fruits have little or no pesticide residue after harvest. Nonorganic papayas are acceptable.
Parsley	✳			Parsley is cultivated like a leafy vegetable, growing close to the ground and sprayed with herbicides and organophosphate pesticides several times during the growth cycle. Organic parsley is the best choice.
Peaches	✳			Peaches are one of the fruits most likely to contain multiple pesticide residues after harvest. Always buy organic. Canned peaches are an acceptable substitute.

FOOD	BUY ORGANIC	NOT ORGANIC	LOCAL	CHEW ON THIS . . .
Peanuts	✳			Peanuts grow underground and are known to absorb toxins from the soil. Buy organic.
Peanut Butter	✳			Organic peanut butter is highly recommended, especially for children.
Pears	✳			Pears are highly likely to contain pesticide residues after harvest. Buy organic, especially for children.
Pecans	✳			If you can find organic pecans, they are a good choice, because pecan trees are often sprayed frequently with pesticides, herbicides, and miticides.
Pineapple		✳		Like most tropical fruits, pineapples have little or no pesticide residue after harvest. Conventionally grown pineapple is acceptable.
Plums	✳		✳	While they test lower than other stone fruits, plums often contain some pesticide residues. Organic is recommended, especially for children.
Poppy Seeds		✳		Poppy plants do not require much, if any, pesticide, although herbicides may be used.

FOOD	BUY ORGANIC	NOT ORGANIC	LOCAL	CHEW ON THIS . . .
Pork			✳	Pork is very difficult to grow organically. Best option is to find a local farmer who raises the animals humanely and talk with him about his philosophy of raising livestock.
Potatoes	✳			Always buy organic. Potatoes, especially Russets, are highly likely to contain multiple pesticide residues. If you cannot find organics, avoid Russet potatoes.
Potato Chips		✳		Potatoes, especially Russets, are highly likely to contain multiple pesticide residues. While little residue is found after processing into chips, organic is best, especially for children.
Pumpkins	✳	✳		Mild pesticides are used on pumpkins early in the growth cycle, although they may be sprayed with herbicides. Fungicide is often sprayed just before harvest. Organic is better for eating, but conventional is fine for jack-o'-lanterns.

FOOD	BUY ORGANIC	NOT ORGANIC	LOCAL	CHEW ON THIS . . .
Radishes		✳		Radishes grow so fast that pests don't have time to do much damage. Nonorganic is acceptable.
Raisins, domestic		✳		Only about 30% of domestic raisins contain pesticide residues, although organic raisins are still the best choice for childen.
Raspberries	✳		✳	Raspberries are highly likely to contain pesticide residue. Always buy organic or pesticide- and fungicide-free local berries.
Rhubarb		✳		Pesticides are almost never used on rhubarb, as the leaves are already highly toxic to many creatures (including humans). Nonorganic rhubarb is a fine choice.
Rice	✳			Buy organic or buy ˙ imported rice. American-grown rice contains 1.4 to 5 times more arsenic on average than rice from Europe, India, and Bangladesh. A likely reason is the American practice of growing rice on defunct cotton fields contaminated with long-banned arsenic pesticides.

FOOD	BUY ORGANIC	NOT ORGANIC	LOCAL	CHEW ON THIS . . .
Salad Greens	✳			Salad greens that grow close to the ground tend to have high pesticide residue levels. Buy organic.
Seafood			✳	Seafood is from a wild system and cannot be certified organic. Avoid farmed fish and prawns, as the fish are fed antibiotics, chicken litter, dyes, and other additives that are not natural in their diet. Obviously, local fish is freshest.
Sesame Seeds		✳		Sesame is sometimes grown in fields contaminated with long-banned arsenic pesticides. Organic is better, but pesticide residues are minor in nonorganic sesame seeds and oils.
Soy Milk	✳			Soy milk is so processed that few pesticide residues remain. However, several very toxic pesticides are used to grow conventional soybeans. Buying organic soy products encourages more organic production, less pollution, and fewer government subsidies. Organic is the best choice for children.

FOOD	BUY ORGANIC	NOT ORGANIC	LOCAL	CHEW ON THIS . . .
Spinach	✳			Always buy organic.
Strawberries	✳			Always buy organic. Avoid giving children strawberries that are conventionally grown.
Sweet Potatoes		✳		Pesticides do not work well for this crop and are used sparingly.
Swiss Chard	✳			Swiss chard is known to pick up toxins and heavy metals from con-taminated soil. The plants also grow close to the ground and tend to have pesticide residues. Buy organic.
Tangerines		✳		Tangerines are among the lowest-ranked citrus fruits for pesticide residues. If you plan to eat the peel, organic is better.
Tea		✳		Chemical pesticides and fertilizers are rarely used on tea plants, because they give an odor and metallic taste to the tea. Free trade tea means the producers pay tea pickers a fair salary.

FOOD	BUY ORGANIC	NOT ORGANIC	LOCAL	CHEW ON THIS . . .
Tofu	✳			Tofu is so processed that few pesticide residues remain. However, several very toxic pesticides are used to grow conventional soybeans. Buying organic tofu encourages more organic soybean production, less pollution, and fewer government subsidies.
Tomatoes			✳	Buy local tomatoes. Always. If you cannot find them, buy whatever tomato smells closest to a homegrown tomato.
Tomato Sauce	✳			Organic tomato products contain more of the cancer-fighting carotenoid lycopene. Choose organic if available.
Turnips	✳			Several toxic pesticides are approved for use on turnip crops. Organic is the best choice.
Watermelons		✳	✳	Pesticides do not work well for this crop and are used sparingly. Local melons will have the best taste.

FOOD	BUY ORGANIC	NOT ORGANIC	LOCAL	CHEW ON THIS . . .
Wheat Flour	✳		`	Not much of the original grain remains after processing, so flours have little pesticide residue.
Wine	✳	✳		Pesticides and fungicides used in wine production pollute the environment and water, but residues are not found in wine. When you find organic wines, buy them.
Winter Squash	✳			Mild pesticides are used on hard winter squashes. Conventionally grown winter squash is coated with an oily wax coating, making the skin inedible. Organic is a better choice, but nonorganic is acceptable if you don't eat the skin.
Yogurt	✳			As with all dairy products, organics allow you to avoid traces of hormones and antibiotics from the cow's milk. Organic is recommended.

FOOD	BUY ORGANIC	NOT ORGANIC	LOCAL	CHEW ON THIS . . .
Zucchini			✳	Zucchini does not tolerate pesticides and herbicides well, but the pesticides that are used on this crop include several toxic organophosphates. Don't you have a neighbor growing zucchini?

• resources •

**Alternative Farming Systems Information Center:
CSA Database**
National Agricultural Library
10301 Baltimore Avenue, Room 132
Beltsville, MD 20705
www.nal.usda.gov/afsic/csa/
Searchable database of CSAs in the United States.

American Community Garden Association
c/o Franklin Park Conservatory
1777 East Broad Street
Columbus, OH 43203
www.communitygarden.org/
*Resources for city dwellers who are interested in finding or starting a
public garden space.*

Boulder Belt Eco-Farm: Lucy Goodman's Blog
http://boulerbelt.blogspot.com/
*Lucy's blog about her farm (Boulder Belt Eco-Farm), sustainable
farming, and her ideas.*

Boulder Belt Eco-Farm

3257 U.S. Route 127 North
Eaton, OH 45320
www.boulderbeltfarm.com/
Sustainable farm featured in the profile on page 6. Boulder Belt Eco-Farm has a CSA and a farm stand, and they sell at the farmers market in uptown Oxford, Ohio, in the Memorial Park.

Canadian Organic Growers

National Office
323 Chapel Street
Ottawa, Ontario K1N 7Z2
www.cog.ca
Canada's national membership-based education and networking organization representing farmers, gardeners, and consumers in all provinces. Includes a listing of organic certification bodies.

Cascade Harvest Coalition

4649 Sunnyside Avenue North, Room 123
Seattle, WA 98103
www.cascadeharvest.org
Organization to promote connections between farmers and the community in Western Washington. Featured in profile on page 39.

The Center for Ecoliteracy

2528 San Pablo Avenue
Berkeley, CA 94702
www.ecoliteracy.org
Dedicated to educating consumers about sustainable living.

Center for Science in the Public Interest

1875 Connecticut Avenue NW, Suite 300
Washington, DC 20009
www.cspinet.org

*An organization that conducts research in health and nutrition. See
their list of ten processed foods you should never eat at
www.cspinet.org/nah/10foods_bad.html. You may also want to
subscribe to their Nutrition Action Healthletter.*

City Farmer/Canada's Office of Urban Agriculture

Box 74567, Kitsilano RPO
Vancouver, BC V6K 4P4
www.cityfarmer.org
*A Canadian site all about urban agriculture, community gardening,
and sustainable agriculture, including rooftop gardens.*

Crescent City Farmers Market of New Orleans

Loyola Twomey Center
7214 St. Charles Avenue, Box 907
New Orleans, LA 70118
www.crescentcityfarmersmarket.org
*See page 141 for a profile of this New Orleans farmers market. Web
site includes recipes, market news, and a calendar of events.*

Diamond Organics

1272 Highway 1
Moss Landing, CA 95039
diamondorganics.com
*Nationwide organic food-delivery service, including produce, baked
goods, and meat.*

Eat Well Guide

www.eatwellguide.org
*A project of Sustainable Table (see page 188), this online directory
includes more than 7,500 farms, stores, restaurants, and other outlets
that offer sustainably raised meat, poultry, dairy, and egg products in
the United States and Canada.*

Eat Wild
29428 129th Avenue SW
Vashon WA 98070
www.eatwild.com
Information about grass-fed food, including a directory of farmers in the United States and Canada. Also sells grass-fed meat, egg, and dairy products.

The Edible Schoolyard
c/o Martin Luther King Jr. Middle School
1781 Rose Street
Berkeley, CA 94703
www.edibleschoolyard.org
Uses lessons learned from the garden and kitchen to promote environmentalism and earth stewardship to schoolchildren.

Environmental Working Group (EWG)
1436 U Street NW, Suite 100
Washington, DC 20009
www.ewg.org
Independent research organization specializing in environmental issues and government policy. The "Shopper's Guide to Pesticides in Produce" and a monthly e-mail bulletin are available through their Web site.

Farmstop
8054 Teasdale Avenue
St. Louis, MO 63130
www.farmstop.com
Agritourism site with links to farm sites across the United States and Canada. If you are looking for a pumpkin patch or winery, this site can help.

FoodRoutes

PO Box 55

35 Apple Lane

Arnot, PA 16911

www.foodroutes.org

A project of the Food Routes Network, this Web site provides news, information, and links "for the food and farming community, community-based nonprofits, the food-concerned public, policy makers and the media."

A Greater Gift

PO Box 365

500 Main Street

New Windsor, MD 21776–0365

www.agreatergift.org

Fair Trade foods, crafts, and gifts from around the world through a nonprofit organization. Artisans and farmers receive up to a 50 percent advance payment so that they can continue to buy raw materials and have a steady income.

Hepworth Farms

1635 RT 9W

Milton, NY, 12547

Sustainable farm featured in the profile on page 28. Hepworth Farms has a CSA, and their products are available at the Park Slope Food Co-op, Whole Foods, and other stores.

Local Harvest

220 21st Avenue

Santa Cruz, CA 95062

www.localharvest.org

Find a farmers' market, family farm, or other source of sustainably grown food in your area of the United States. More than nine thousand members are listed through this informational resource.

Madison Market (Central Co-op)

1600 East Madison Street
Seattle, WA 98122
www.madisonmarket.com
I shop at this natural food co-op in Seattle's Capitol Hill neighborhood, and they are indirectly mentioned in this book many times. Lots of cool tattoos on the checkout clerks, and a very knowledgeable staff.

Molecular Expressions: The Pesticide Collection

www.microscopy.fsu.edu/pesticides
Pesticides are a depressing topic, but this Florida State University site shows images of more than common pesticides that were recrystallized and photographed under a microscope with the goal of demonstrating "the irony between the beautiful patterns generated by crystallized pesticides and the dangerous nature of their mechanism of action."

National Organic Standards Board

c/o National Organic Program
1400 Independence Avenue SW, Room 2510
South Building
Washington, DC 20250
http://www.ams.usda.gov/nosb/
The NOSB assists the secretary of agriculture to develop standards for substances to be used in organic production. The board takes public comments on proposed changes to organic standards.

New American Dream

6930 Carroll Avenue, Suite 900
Takoma Park, MD 20912
www.newdream.org
Resources for consumers to use buying power to create positive change.

The New Farm

www.newfarm.org

Run by the Rodale Institute, this site has a discussion board where sustainable or organic farmers and wanna-be organic farmers can discuss issues and problem-solve.

Niman Ranch

1025 E. 12th Street

Oakland, CA 94606

www.nimanranch.com

Antibiotic- and hormone-free beef, lamb, and pork products, including Fearless Franks (hot dogs made from high-quality beef and pork cuts that even come in an uncured version for kids).

Organic Consumers Association

6771 South Silver Hill Drive

Finland, MN 55603

www.organicconsumers.org

This grassroots nonprofit organization campaigns for "health, justice, and sustainability." See their list of CSAs compiled by state at http://www.organicconsumers.org/csa.htm.

Organic Valley Family of Farms

CROPP Cooperative

One Organic Way

LaFarge, WI 54639

http://organicvalley.coop

An organic farming cooperative of more than eight hundred family farms. Site includes information on organic foods as well as recipes and a search feature to find online retailers or retailers in your area.

PANNA (Pesticide Action Network North America)
49 Powell Street, Suite 500
San Francisco, CA 94102
http://panna.org/
Antipesticide activism and information about pesticides and human health.

Park Slope Food Co-op
782 Union Street
Brooklyn, NY 11215
http://foodcoop.com
With more than twelve thousand members, this co-op is located between 6th and 7th Avenues in Brooklyn. Produce buyer Allen Zimmerman is featured in the profile on page 59. Web site includes recipes that use organic foods.

Pesticide Action Network Pesticide Database
www.pesticideinfo.org
Search for toxicity and regulatory information on hundreds of pesticides, insecticides, and herbicides at this PANNA Web site.

Petaluma Poultry
PO Box 7368
2700 Lakeville Highway
Petaluma, CA 94955
www.petalumapoultry.com
Provides information about sustainability and organic and free-range poultry, including brand names Rosie Organic Free Range Chicken (the first chicken in the United States to be certified organic) and Rocky Range Chicken. Also includes recipes for poultry and a variety of other meats.

PCC (Puget Consumers Co-op)
4201 Roosevelt Way NE
Seattle, WA 98105
www.pccnaturalmarkets.com
Seattle-area organic and natural foods market. Web site includes recipes as well as information on organics, farmland preservation, genetically engineered foods, irradiated foods, mad cow, and sustainable seafood.

Purity Organics
14900 West Belmont Avenue
Kerman, California 93630
www.purityorganics.com
Small cooperative that grows organic almonds. One of the few Internet sources for organic almonds.

The Rodale Institute
611 Siegfriedale Road
Kutztown, PA 19530–9320
www.rodaleinstitute.org
Learn about healthy soil, pesticide-free farming, and agricultural education. This site also includes a farm locator to help consumers, farmers, and others find farm services in their area.

Sea Breeze Farm
10730 SW 116th Street
Vashon Island, WA 98070
http://home.comcast.net/~georgepage2/Index.html
Sustainable farm featured in the profile on page 74. This grass-based animal farm produces meats (beef, ducks, pork, and chicken), dairy products, and eggs, and is also home to Sweetbread Cellars winery (http://sweetbreadcellars.com/).

Slow Food
http://slowfood.com

Slow Food USA National Office
20 Jay Street, Suite 313
Brooklyn, NY 11201
www.slowfoodusa.org
Global organization that provides support for traditional foods, farm-
ing, and biodiversity. Now with more than eighty thousand members,
Slow Food was founded in 1989 "to counteract fast food and fast life,
the disappearance of local food traditions and people's dwindling
interest in the food they eat, where it comes from, how it tastes and how
our food choices affect the rest of the world."

Small Potatoes Urban Delivery (Spuds)
1660 E. Hastings Street
Vancouver, BC, V5L 1S6
www.spud.com
Organic and local grocery delivery service in Vancouver and Victoria,
British Columbia; Calgary, Alberta, and other Canadian locations.
Also delivers in northwestern Washington, including Seattle. More than
half of Spud's products are from local sources.

The Sustainable Table
215 Lexington Avenue, Suite 1001
New York, NY 10016
http://sustainabletable.org
Understand sustainable food and shopping along with other food-
related issues. Web site includes shopping guides and the Eat Well Guide
to sources of sustainable meat, poultry, dairy, and eggs in the United
States and Canada.

Urban Gardening Help

www.urbangardeninghelp.com

Tips and advice on planning an urban garden and growing your own food. Also includes information on community gardens and CSAs.

USDA (farmers markets listed by state)

www.ams.usda.gov/farmersmarkets/map.htm

Find a farmers market in your area on this Web site from the USDA's Agricultural Marketing Service branch.

Whistling Train Farm

27112 78th Avenue South

Kent, WA 98032

www.whistlingtrainfarm.com

Sustainable farm featured in the profile on page 117. Whistling Train Farm has a CSA and sells at the University District and the West Seattle farmers' markets. Lots of yummy recipes at their "How to Eat It" page.

Wild Oats Natural Markets

3375 Mitchell Lane

Boulder, CO 80301

www.wildoats.com

Information about the Wild Oats philosophy, buying practices, products, and store locations. Also includes recipes, even for special diets such as low-carb, dairy free, gluten free, and vegan.

Whole Foods Market

www.wholefoodsmarket.com

Information about the Whole Foods philosophy, store locations, products, and events. Includes recipes along with information on health and nutrition as well as food-related issues.

• endnotes •

Chapter 1

1. "Organic2006: Consumer Attitudes and Behavior Five Years Later and into the Future, " report from the Hartman Group, Inc., May 2006.
2. Ann Zimmerman, "Planting the Seeds: Big Food Companies Sell More Organic Products, But Production Is Risky," *Wall Street Journal*, August 23, 2006, B-1.
3. "NBJ's Healthy Foods Report 2006," *Nutrition Business Journal*, October 1, 2006, sec. 1.
4. "Organic2006."
5. Ibid.
6. Libby Quaid, "More than Grass Is on Menu for Grass-Fed Cattle," *Seattle Post-Intelligencer*, September 4, 2006, sec. A. Available online at http://seattlepi.nwsource.com/national/283698_beef04.html.
7. Allen Zimmerman, interview by the author, October 3, 2006.
8. Steven Shapin, "Paradise Sold: What Are You Buying When You Buy Organic?" *The New Yorker*, May 15, 2006, 86. Available online at www.newyorker.com/critics/atlarge/articles/060515crat_atlarge.
9. Eric Schlosser, *Fast Food Nation: The Dark Side of the All-American Meal*, by (Boston: Houghton Mifflin, 2001).
10. Shapin, "Paradise Sold."
11. "Organic2006."("Almost three-quarters [73%] of the U.S. population consume organic foods or beverages at least occasionally.")

Chapter 2

1. Theo Colborn, Dianne Dumanoski, and John Peterson Myers, *Our Stolen Future: Are We Threatening Our Fertility, Intelligence, and Survival? A Scientific Detective Story* (New York: Dutton, 1996).

2. BBC News website, "DDT 'link' to slow child progress," Wednesday, 5 July 2006. Available online at http://news.bbc.co.uk/1/hi/health/5145450.stm.

3. "Organics—Frequently Asked Questions, 'Are organic foods healthier?'" Whole Foods Market Web site (http://www.wholefoodsmarket.com/issues/organic/faq.html)

4. PBS, *Frontline*, "Fooling with Nature," interview with Fredrick Vom Saal, PhD, originally aired June 2, 1998. Transcript available online at http://www.pbs.org/wgbh/pages/frontline/shows/nature/interviews/vomsaal.html

5. W. V. Welshons, S. C. Nagel. K. A. Thayer, B. M. Judy, and F. S. vom Saal. 1999. "Low-dose Bioactivity of Xenoestrogens in Animals: Fetal Exposure to Low Doses of Methoxychlor and Other Xenoestrogens Increases adult Prostate Size in Mice." *Toxicology and Industrial Health* 15:12—25.

6. Environmental Working Group, "Body Burden—The Pollution in Newborns: A Benchmark Investigation of Industrial Chemicals, Pollutants, and Pesticides in Umbilical Cord Blood," July 14, 2005 Environmental Working Group Web site (http://www.ewg.org/reports/bodbyburden2/).

7 Gertrud S. Berkowitz, James G. Wetmur, Elena Birman-Deych, Josephine Obel, et al., "In Utero Pesticide Exposure, Maternal Paraoxonase Activity, and Head Circumference," *Environmental Health Perspectives* 112, no. 3 (March 2004), 388—91.

8. Richard A. Fenske, "Children's Pesticide Exposure in the Seattle Metropolitan Area," *Agrichemical and Environmental News* 190 (February 2002), 4. Available online at http://www.aenews.wsu.edu/Feb02AENews/Fenske/FenskePDF.pdf.

9. R. A. Fenske, G. Kedan, C. Lu, J. A. Fisker-Andersen, and C. L. Curl. "Assessment of Organophosphorus Pesticide Exposures in the Diets of Preschool Children in Washington State," *Journal of Exposure Analalysis and Environmental Epidemiology* 12, no. 1 (2002), 21—28.

10. Colburn, "Our Stolen Future."

11. Richard Fagerlund, "Pesticides' Inert Ingredients Should Also Cause Concern," *San Francisco Chronicle*, April 22, 2006, F-2. Available online at http://www.sfgate.com/cgi-bin/article.cgi?f=/c/a/2006/04/22/hogugicb0d1.dtl.

12. Warren Cornwall, "Pesticide Exec to Lead Regional EPA Office," *Seattle Times*, October 7, 2006, sec. B.

13. The letter is available online at http://www.panna.org/resources/documents/epaScientistsFqpa.pdf.

Chapter 3

1. Berkowitz et al. "In Utero Pesticide Exposure, Maternal Paraoxonase Activity, and Head Circumference."

2. "Chlorpyrifos Factsheet, Part 2: Human Exposure," *Journal of Pesticide Reform* 15, Number 1, Spring 1995. Northwest Coalition for Alternatives to Pesticides, Eugene, OR.

3. Rodale Institute Web site, History page (http://www.rodaleinstitute .org/about/where_set.html).

4. Rachel Carson, *Silent Spring* (Boston: Houghton Mifflin, 1962).

5. Rachel Carson's obituary, published October 15, 1964 in the *The New York Times*. Available online at http://www.nytimes.com/books/97/10/05/reviews/carson-obit.html?_r=1&oref=slogin

6. Robert Rodale, testimony. New York State public hearing in the matter of organic foods. New York City, December 1, 1972.

Chapter 4

1. "Organic2006."

2. *The World of Organic Agriculture: Statistics and Emerging Trends 2004*; published by the International Federation of Organic Agriculture Movements (IFOAM), es. Helga Willer and Minou Yussefi, 21. Available online at http://www.soel.de/inhalte/publikationen/s/s_74.pdf.

3. Zimmerman, "Planting the Seeds."

4. *The World of Organic Agriculture 2004*.

5. Zimmerman, "Planting the Seeds."

6. Josee Rose, "Soaring Sales of Organic Foods Squeeze Supermarket Suppliers," *Wall Street Journal*, August 30, 2006, A-8.

7. Rose, "Soaring Sales of Organic Foods."

8. Zimmerman, "Planting the Seeds."

9. The Organic Farming Research Organization Web site at http://ofrf.org/resources/organicfaqs.html.

10. International Federation of Organic Agriculture Movements (IFOAM), "The World of Organic Agriculture: More Than 31 Million Hectares Worldwide," IFOAM Web site (http://www.ifoam.org/press/press/Statistics_2006.html), February 14, 2006.

11. Paula Lavigne, "Is Organic Food the Real Deal?" *Dallas Morning News*, July 17, 2006, sec. A. Available online at http://www.dallasnews.com/sharedcontent/dws/dn/latestnews/stories/071606dncco organics.19c550e.html.

12. *World of Organic Agriculture*, 2004.

13. Allen Zimmerman, interview by the author, October 3, 2006.

14. Lavigne, "Is Organic Food the Real Deal?"

15. USDA Web site.

16. Andrew Martin, "Critics Say Dairy Tests the Boundaries and Spirit of What 'Organic' Means," *Chicago Tribune*, August 20, 2006, 1.

17. Katy McLaughlin, "At the Market: A New Twist in the Organic Milk Debate," *Wall Street Journal* (Eastern edition), December 10, 2005, P-14. Available online at http://www.organicconsumers.org/rBGH/milk121905.cfm.htm.

18. Lucy Goodman, interview by the author, March 18, 2006.

Chapter 5

1. "Uncle Sam's Teat: Can America's Farmers Be Weaned from Their Government Money?" *Economist*, September 7, 2006. Available online at http://www.economist.com/world/na/displaystory.cfm?story_id=7887994.

2. Environmental Working Group, Farm Subsidy Database, Environmental Working Group Web site. Available online at http://www.ewg.org:16080/farm/whatsnew_introduction.php

3. Ibid.

Chapter 6

1. Andrew Weil, *8 Weeks to Optimal Health: A Proven Program for Taking Full Advantage of Your Body's Natural Healing Power*, rev. ed. (New York: Knopf, 2006).
2. Environmental Working Group, "EWG in the News: U.S.: High Pesticide Level Marks 'Dirty Dozen' Fruits, Vegetables," October 19, 2006, http://www.ewg.org/news/story.php?id=5557. Also see www.foodnews.org for a more complete listing.

Chapter 7

1. Peter Reinhart, *American Pie: My Search for the Perfect Pizza* (Berkeley, CA: Ten Speed Press, 2003.
2. United States Food and Drug Administration fact sheet, "Nationwide E. Coli 0157:H7 Outbreak: Questions & Answers"October 20, 2006. Available online at http://www.cfsan.fda.gov/~dms/spinacqa.html.
3. Yutaka Iwata, F. A. Gunther, and W. E. Westlake, "Uptake of a PCB (Aroclor 1254) from Soil by Carrots under Field Conditions;" *Bulletin of Environmental Contamination and Toxicology* 11, no. 6 (June 1974), 523–28.
4. Guy Clark, "Homegrown Tomatoes," from the live album *Keepers*, Sugar Hill Records SHCD-1055, 1997.
5. Ruth Yaron, *Super Baby Food: A Fast, Easy, Economical Method of Making Super Healthy Homemade Baby Food for Your Super Baby* (Archbald, PA: F. J. Roberts, 1997).
6. "Opinion of the Scientific Committee on Veterinary Measures Relating to Public Health: Review of Previous SCVPH Opinions of 30 April 1999 and 3 May 2000 on the Potential Risks to Human Health from Hormone Residues from Bovine Meat and meat Products," European Commission, Health and Consumer Directorate, April 10, 2002.
7. Quoted from CBS News, "Link Eyed Between Beef and Cancer," *CBS News Online*, May 20, 2003. Available at http://www.cbsnews.com/stories/2003/05/20/eveningnews/main554857.shtml.
8. FDA Press Release, 2005, "FDA Proposes Additional 'Mad Cow' Safeguards," October 4. Available online at http://www.fda.gov/bbs/topics/news/2005/new01240.html.

9. University of Missouri Extension Web site, "G2077, Feeding Poultry Litter to Beef Cattle," pub. October 2005. Available online at http://muextension.missouri.edu/explore/agguides/ansci/g02077.htm.

10. Jo Robinson, *Why Grassfed Is Best! The Surprising Benefits of Grassfed Meats, Eggs, and Dairy Products* (Vashon, WA: Vashon Island Press, 2000).

11. Michael F. Jacobson, *Six Arguments for a Greener Diet: How a More Plant-Based Diet Could Save Your Health and the Environment*, Center for Science in the Public Interest, August 2006, 67.

12. Tamar Lasky, Wenyu Sun, Abdel Kadry, and Michael K. Hoffman, "Mean Total Arsenic Concentrations in Chicken 1989–2000 and Estimated Exposures for Consumers of Chicken," Office of Public Health and Science, Food Safety and Inspection Service, U.S. Department of Agriculture, reported in *Environmental Health Perspectives* 112, no. 1 (January 2004), 18–21.

13. David Wallinga, *Playing Chicken: Avoiding Arsenic in Your Meat, Institute for Agriculture and Trade Policy*, Food and Health Program, April 2006. Available online at http://www.environmentalobservatory.org/library.cfm?refid=80529

14. Ronald C. Kaltreider, Alisa M. Davis, Jean P. Lariviere, and Joshua W. Hamilton, "Arsenic Alters the Function of the Glucocorticoid Receptor as a Transcription Factor," *Environmental Health Perspectives* 109, no. 3 (2001), 245–51. Available online at http://www.ehponline.org/docs/2001/109p245–251kaltreider/abstract.html.

15. McLaughlin, "At the Market: A New Twist In the Organic Milk Debate."

16. Ibid.

17. Michael D. Lemonick, "Teens Before Their Time," *Time*, October 30, 2000. Available online at http://www.time.com/time/magazine/article/0,9171,998347,00.html.

18. Gary Steinman, "Mechanisms of Twinning: VII. Effect of Diet and Heredity on the Human Twinning Rate," *Journal of Reproductive Medicine* 51, no. 5 (May 2006), 405–10.

19. O. I. Kalantzi, K. C. Jones, R. E. Alcock, P. A. Johnston, et al., "The Global Distribution of PCBs and Organochlorine Pesticides in Butter," *Environmental Science and Technology* 35, no. 6 (March 2001), 1013–18.

ENDNOTES

• • • • • • •

20. National Organic Standards Board, Aquatic Animal Task Force, "Recommendation on Operations that Produce Aquatic Animals," May 30, 2001.

21. P. N. Williams, A. H. Price, A. Raab, et al. "Variation in Arsenic Speciation and Concentration in Paddy Rice Related to Dietary Exposure, *Environmental Science and Technology* 39, no. 15 (2005), 5531–40. Available online at http://pubs.acs.org/cgi-bin/sample.cgi/esthag/2005/39/i15/pdf/es0502324.pdf.

Chapter 8

1. Ben Hoyt, sustainable farmer, Alm Hill Gardens, interview with author, May 2006, Everson, Washington.

2. According to the Co-op Directory Listing, available online at http://www.coopdirectory.org/directory.htm.

3. USDA, "Farmers Market Growth," USDA Web site, http://www.ams.usda.gov/farmersmarkets/FarmersMarketGrowth.htm.

• glossary •

ACETYLCHOLINE: A small molecule that flows from nerve endings. Some pesticides operate by preventing the breakdown of acetylcholine, which causes overstimulation, leading to intense spasms of the muscles, including the heart.

AGRIBUSINESS: Farming on a large scale, including those businesses associated with the production, processing, and distribution of agricultural products.

ALGAECIDES: Chemicals used to kill algae.

ALLICIN: A powerful antifungal compound obtained from garlic cloves, which also have insect repellant properties.

ANDROGENS: A compound, generally a hormone, that stimulates the development of male characteristics. Testosterone is the primary androgen, but steroid hormones are also androgens.

AQUACULTURE: The cultivation of fish, shellfish and other water-dwelling creatures. Catfish, tilapia, salmon, prawns, and mussels are often raised on fish "farms."

ARC OF TASTE: The Slow Food organization defines this term as traditional foods that are threatened by modern methods. Slow Food contends that standardization and mass production produces low-quality food with a high environmental cost.

BACILLUS THURINGIENSIS (BT): This microorganism is toxic to members of the caterpillar family, but does not harm other insects. Bt is considered an environmentally friendly way to control certain pests.

BLIGHT: Plant diseases that manifest as sudden wilting and dying of affected plants, especially young plants. Potatoes are susceptible to blight.

BOVINE SPONGIFORM ENCEPHALOPATHY (BSE): *See mad cow disease.*

BROAD-SPECTRUM INSECTICIDES: Pesticides that are toxic to a wide variety of insects, including many beneficial insects, such as honeybees, ladybugs and other predatory insects.

CALIFORNIA CERTIFIED ORGANIC FARMERS (CCOF): Founded in 1973, CCOF helped create the original organic standards. Today, it is one of the oldest and largest organic certification and trade associations in California.

CARBAMATES: Pesticides such as sevin, aldicarb, and carbaryl, often used on fruit crops. Exposure has been linked with hormonal changes, DNA damage, birth defects, and abnormal sperm, ovaries, and eggs.

CARCINOGENIC: Capable of causing cancer.

CHLORINATED HYDROCARBONS: DDT, aldrin, endrin, and chlordane are included in this category. The EPA banned many chlorinated hydrocarbons from use in the United States during the 1970s and '80s, because these insecticides persist in the environment and build up in the fatty tissues of humans and animals.

CHLOROTHALONIL: An active and inert ingredient in pesticides that is considered a probable human carcinogen.

CHOLINESTERASE: An enzyme produced in the liver. The poisonous effects of organophosphorous and carbamate pesticides inhibit cholinesterase.

CLEAN AIR ACT: A series of EPA initiatives designed to reduce air pollution, toxic emissions, and acid rain within the United States.

CSA: Community supported agriculture; typically a purchased share in a small farm that provides the customer with a box of mixed produce each week. Members of CSAs share the risks and benefits of food production.

DAP: Dialkyl phosphate. The breakdown product of DDT, which is secreted in urine samples.

DDT: Dichloro-diphenyl-trichloroethane. The first modern and best-known pesticide. Originally developed as an insecticide during in World War II to combat mosquitoes, DDT was finally banned in 1972 because it causes cancer in humans and animals.

DIRTY DOZEN: A list of the twelve foods most likely to contain pesticide residue created by the Environmental Working Group from data published by the USDA.

ENDOCRINE DISRUPTORS: Chemicals that mimic or inhibit the effects of hormones in the bodies of humans and animals.

ENDOSULFAN: A pesticide that affects the function of the central nervous system.

EPA: Environmental Protection Agency.

ENVIRONMENTAL WORKING GROUP (EWG): A nonprofit environmental research organization and government watchdog group based in Washington, D.C. The EWG provides information to consumers about pesticides, food production and farm policy, along with other environmental issues.

ETHICAL EATERS: People who make decisions about how and why they buy food based fully or partially on their hope that those food choices can positively impact farming practices. Some examples of those foods are Fair Trade chocolate, shade-grown coffee, free-range chickens, organic or sustainably farmed foods, and grass-fed beef.

FAIR TRADE CERTIFIED: Products that have been inspected and verified by a Fair Trade certification organization. The label indicates that the people who produce your coffee, tea, cocoa, chocolate, spices, sugar, rice, and vanilla are paid a fair price, and receive other economic and social benefits.

FARM SUBSIDIES: Payments from the government to farmers who grow certain commodity crops, such as corn, wheat, soybeans, cotton, and rice. Subsidies are controversial because they give large-scale farmers an unfair competitive advantage and suppress the prices of commodities.

FDA: Food and Drug Administration.

FEDERAL INSECTICIDE, FUNGICIDE, AND RODENTICIDE ACT OF 1972: The federal law which set up the U.S. system of pesticide regulation. The law is administered by the EPA and the appropriate environmental agencies of each state. FIFRA created the registration process for pesticides. Registration is done after data is collected to determine the effectiveness, the intended use, the appropriate dosage, and the hazards of a pesticide.

FOOD QUALITY PROTECTION ACT (FQPA): Passed by Congress in 1996, FQPA mandates updated standards for all pesticides used on food, provides special protections against pesticide exposure for children, and creates incentives for developing crop protection tools for farmers. The Act also requires periodic reevaluation of pesticide registrations and tolerances.

FUMIGANT: A chemical compound used as a disinfectant or pesticide.

GMO (GENETICALLY MODIFIED ORGANISM): A plant created through genetic engineering. The most widely grown GMO crops are soybeans, corn, canola (rapeseed), and cotton. Most GMOs are either "insect-resistant" or "herbicide-tolerant" crops. The insect-resistant crops produce a toxin as they grow, in every cell of the plant, throughout the entire growth cycle.

HDL CHOLESTEROL: High-density lipoprotein, also known as the "good" cholesterol because high levels seem to have a protective effect against heart disease and heart attacks.

HEAVY METALS: Any metallic chemical element that has a relatively high density and is toxic, highly toxic, or poisonous at low concentrations. Heavy metals include mercury, cadmium, arsenic, chromium, thallium, and lead.

HORMONE GROWTH PROMOTANTS (HGPS): Hormones implanted or injected into cattle to increase milk production or bulk up beef cattle. Few countries other than the U.S. and Canada have approved the use of HGPs, while many others, such as countries in the EU, have banned their use.

MAD COW DISEASE: Bovine spongiform encepholopathy (BSE) is a fatal neurological disease that affects cattle. Symptoms of the disease include an unsteady gait, excitability, and dementia. When transmitted to humans, the disease is called Creutzfeldt-Jakob disease, and results in dementia and death.

MALATHION: An broad-spectrum pesticide used on agricultural crops, as well as to kill head lice, fleas, and mosquitos.

MANURE POOLS: On factory farms, crating or housing animals in pens with slotted floors allows large quantities of manure to build up. The manure is often pumped into large, smelly lagoons that sometimes overflow during heavy rains or floods.

MEFENOXAM: A fungicide used on carrots, strawberries, spinach, and other crops. Mefenoxam is also used on nonorganic seeds.

METHYL BROMIDE: A broad-spectrum pesticide used to control insects, weeds, rodents, and pathogens. A colorless, odorless gas at room temperature, methyl bromide is normally applied as a liquid under pressure that vaporizes upon release at the point of application. The use of methyl bromide as a pesticide is currently being phased out both in the United States and all other countries.

MILDECIDES: Chemicals that prevent or eliminate mildew from food crops.

MONOCULTURE: The practice of growing a single crop.

MONTREAL PROTOCOL: An international agreement designed to protect the ozone layer by phasing out the production and consumption of compounds that are known to deplete ozone.

MUTAGENS: A chemical compound that creates mutations. Most mutagens are also carcinogens.

NATIONAL AGRICULTURAL STATISTICS SERVICE (NASS) NATIONAL ORGANIC PROGRAM (NOP): Passed in 1990, the NOP requires the USDA to develop consistent, nationwide standards and labels for organic foods to benefit consumers.

NATIONAL ORGANIC STANDARDS BOARD (NOSB): The board assists the U.S. Secretary of Agriculture in developing standards for any substance used for organic production.

NEMATICIDES: A chemical used for killing nematodes that are parasitic to plants.

NEMATODES: Nematodes are small wormlike creatures that live in soil. Many nematodes are parasites of plants or animals.

NEURON: Nerve cells that process information in the central nervous system or humans and animals.

NEUROTOXIN: A toxin that acts specifically on the nerve cells.

NOP STANDARDS: In 2002 the USDA adopted a set of national standards that food labeled "organic" must meet, whether it is grown in the United States or imported from other countries.

OMEGA-3 FATTY ACIDS: Fatty acids that are essential to human health but cannot be made by the body. They must be obtained from food and are primarily found in fish and certain plant oils. Extensive research has found that omega-3 fatty acids increase cognitive function, reduce inflammation, and help prevent heart disease and arthritis

ORGANIC FOODS PRODUCTION ACT (OFPA): The act establishes uniform national standards for the production and handling of foods that are labeled as "organic." The OFPA sets the certification standards for the organic certification process.

ORGANOPHOSPHATE: Organophosphates are a diverse group of chemicals containing phosphorus used in agriculture, residential areas, and industry. Examples of organophosphates include insecticides (malathion, parathion, diazinon, fenthion, dichlorvos, chlorpyrifos) and nerve gases, among others.

PCBS: Polychlorinated biphenyls. A class of endocrine-disrupting chemical compounds found in many plastics and pesticides that are harmful to humans.

PERMETHRIN: An neurotoxin insecticide widely used on cotton, wheat, corn, alfalfa, and other crops. Laboratory tests suggest that permethrin is especially toxic for children. The EPA classifies permethrin as a carcinogen because it causes lung tumors in female mice and liver tumors in mice of both sexes. In laboratory tests, permethrin inhibits the immune system and causes chromosome aberrations in human cells.

PERSISTENT ORGANIC POLLUTANTS (POP): Long-lasting, toxic chemicals in the environment. They are primarily products and by-products from pesticides, industrial processes, and chemical manufacturing. POPs accumulate in the body fat of humans, marine mammals, and other animals, and are passed from mother to fetus. They also travel long distances on wind and water currents. Even tiny quantities of POPs cause nervous system damage, diseases of the immune system, reproductive disorders, and cancer.

PESTICIDE DATA PROGRAM (PDP): The USDA's Pesticide Data Program focuses its testing on fruits and vegetables that have been identified by the EPA as having set pesticide tolerances.

RBGH AND RBST GROWTH HORMONES: Also known as "crack" for cows, these hormones "rev up" a cow's body, forcing it to produce a greater volume of milk. However, it also makes them sick. According to the FDA, cows injected with rBGH suffer from increased udder infections (mastitis), reproductive problems, digestive disorders, foot ailments, and persistent sores. These health problems are in turn treated with antibiotic injections.

SAMPLING: The process of collecting and testing random samples of food for pesticides and other contaminants. The foods used for sampling are a very small percentage of the total food produced each year, but they are intended to represent fresh foods that are commonly available to the American consumer.

SCALE: Insects that attack plants. They appear as flat or slightly mounded waxy, brown scales on affected leaves and stems. The insect under the protective scale feeds on plant sap and can transmit diseases.

SEWAGE SLUDGE: Anything flushed, poured, or dumped into our massive wastewater system. The sludge sprayed on food crop fields is a dangerous blend of heavy metals, industrial by-products, bacteria, drug residues, and radioactive materials.

SLOW FOOD CONVIVIUM: A group that celebrates the joy of food and works to preserve traditional foods and methods of preparation. Conviviums started to appear in the UK and other parts of the world during the late 1990s to refer to local local chapters of the Slow Food movement.

SUSTAINABILITY: Methods of growing, harvesting, and using agricultural products and resources so that they are not depleted or permanently damaged. The overriding philosophy is that using a resource in the present should not prevent future generations from using that resource.

SYNAPSE: The synapse is a small gap between neurons where information from one neuron flows to another neuron.

TOXICITY CATEGORY I COMPOUND: The EPA's highest toxicity category, reserved for the most deadly substances.

TRANSITIONAL ORGANIC: Food grown on land that has not yet met the three-year chemical free criteria to be considered for organic certification.

USDA: United States Department of Agriculture.

XENOESTROGEN: Imitating or increasing the effect of estrogen.

• acknowledgments •

I'd like to thank the following people for their help with this book:

Matthew Lore, my publisher, for nurturing this book and for providing me with a forum to explore this dynamic and exciting topic.

Jill Hughes, copy editor, for her many good catches and helpful suggestions.

George Page, Shelley Verdi, Mike Pasco, Amy Hepworth and Lucy Goodman, the dedicated farmers who educated me not only about farming but about the passion that truly great farmers feel about their land. These people love their farms, and they are truly inspiring stewards of that land.

Poppy Tooker, a New Orleans phenomenon, for saving the Cresent City Farmers' Market and for telling me her story.

Mary Embleton of Cascade Harvest Coalition, for sharing her enthusiasm and philosophy about the value of agriculture and community.

Allen Zimmerman of the Park Slope Food Co-op, who allowed me to tap his remarkable knowledge of natural and organic produce. His experiences with garlic from China led me to explore the ways that big business is changing the face of organics.

The farmers at the West Seattle Farmers' Market, who show up every Sunday, rain or shine, with smiles, hot cider, pastries, and piles of fresh food for all of their customers.

Kim Severson of the *New York Times,* for her unwavering support and for Poppy's phone number.

Allison Burke, my little daughter, whose energy and love keeps me alive.

Pat Burke, my wife, who never lost her enthusiasm for this book or for me. Thanks to her I am healthy, happy, and warm, and I love her for it.

My friends, neighbors and family, who were always happy to play with my daughter so I could work on this book.

• index •

INDEX
· · · · · ·

grapes, 89, 100, 165–66
grass-fed beef, 111–12
Greater Gift, A, 183
green beans, 105–6, 166
green onions, 104–5, 166
grocery chains, 11, 33, 52, 147. *See also*
    corporatization of organic farming;
    specific stores

Harvest Celebration, 39–40
HDL cholesterol (high-density
    lipoprotein), 202–3
health
    eating for, 155
    quality of life and, xiv–xv
    transitioning to healthier eating,
        78–79, 149–50, 155
    See also pesticide exposure and
        health
heavy metals
    about, 203
    in beets, 132
    in carrots, 91, 94, 103, 161
    in humans, 19
    in leafy vegetables, 102, 175
    in peanuts, 91
    in rice, 132
    See also arsenic
heirloom varietals, 145
Hepworth, Amy, 28–30, 55
Hepworth Farms, 28–30, 183
herbicides, 17–18, 115–19
hippies, 43–44
home-delivery services, 146–47
Horizon Organics, 10, 57
hormonal signaling disruptors,
    17–18
hormone growth promotants (HGPS),
    109–10, 122–23, 203
hormones and reproductive system
    development, 23
humane slaughter, 118
Hurricane Katrina, 141–44

inert ingredients in pesticides, 26
infants, 16–17, 23–24, 98–99
insects and monoculture, 37
Institute for Agriculture and Trade
    Policy, 113
insulin-like growth factor, 123
International Fairtrade Certification
    Mark, 71
International Federation of Alterna-
    tive Trade, 71

Johnson, Stephen, 31–32
juice, 166, 170

kale, 102, 166
Katrina, 141–44
Kennedy, John F., 42
ketchup, 167
kiwi, on Clean Fifteen list, 92
Kroger Company, 11, 52

labeling of produce, 33
lead. *See* heavy metals
leafy vegetables, 101–3. *See also specific*
    vegetables
leeks, 104–5, 167
lemons, 167
lettuce, 101–3, 167
limes, 167
lobbyists of agribusiness companies,
    xiv, 14, 31–33, 110
local and sustainable
    added value of, 62, 64
    environmental costs of shipping,
        68
    values related to, 65, 66, 79–81
    Whistling Train Farm, 115–19,
        189
Local Harvest, 183
locally grown food, definition of,
    68–69
local sources, importance of
    about, 33–34, 58, 189

INDEX

transitional organics, 53, 69–70, 207
tropical fruits, 101
trust issues, 11–12
turnips, 176
twins, increasing number of, 122–23

union reps for EPA scientists, 31–32
United Kingdom's organic standards, 45
U-pick, 139–40
Urban Gardening Help, 189
USDA (United States Department of Agriculture)
    on arsenic levels in chicken meat, 113
    monitoring and communicating with, 34
    on pesticide-levels, 3, 84–85
    role of, 27
    sustainable farmer's opinion of, 5
    See also certified organic label; EPA; FDA

values
    businesses' awareness of, 63–64, 66
    convenience versus, 12
    personal awareness of, 64, 153
    of Rodale, 38
    traditional values of organic farming, 65
    utilizing for cost-benefit analysis, 79–81
    See also local and sustainable
vegan diets, 122–23
vegetables, 101–7, 164, 176

See also specific vegetables
Verdi, Mike, 115–19
vinclozolin, 17–18
vine fruits, 100
vom Saal, Frederick, 19, 23–24

Wall Street Journal, 52
Wal-Mart, 11, 52, 54, 56, 65–66, 148
watermelons, 92, 100, 176
wheat flour, 132–33, 177
Whistling Train Farm, 115–19, 189
Whole Foods Markets
    about, 136–37, 189
    Chinese produce and, 54, 56
    meats from, 112, 114
    organic product line, 11, 52
    small farmers and, 138
Wild Oats Natural Markets, 112, 114, 136–38, 189
wine, 177
winter squash, 107–8, 177
World War II, 36, 37
worldwide shipping, environmental costs of, 55–56

xenoestrogenic chemicals, 17–18, 88, 207

Yaron, Ruth, 98
yogurt, 177

Zeranol, 109
Zimmerman, Allen, 54, 59–62
zucchini, 177